PRINCI
COLONIC I

IN THE SAME SERIES:

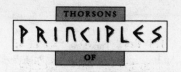

COLONIC IRRIGATION

JILLIE COLLINGS

Thorsons
An Imprint of HarperCollinsPublishers

Thorsons
An Imprint of HarperCollins*Publishers*
77–85 Fulham Palace Road
Hammersmith, London W6 8JB
1160 Battery Street
San Francisco, California 94111–1213

Published by Thorsons 1996

1 3 5 7 9 10 8 6 4 2

A catalogue record for this book
is available from the British Library

ISBN 0 7225 3029 3

Printed in Great Britain by
HarperCollinsManufacturing Glasgow

THE PUBLISHERS WOULD LIKE TO THANK
JILLIE COLLINGS FOR HER SUGGESTION FOR THE TITLE
OF THIS SERIES, PRINCIPLES OF . . .

CONTENTS

INTRODUCTION

There can be no other therapy which is more misunderstood, maligned and misused (by some) than colonic irrigation, to give it its original name – though it is more frequently known today as colonic hydrotherapy or colon therapy. Basically, it is a method whereby purified water is introduced into the colon through a specially sterilized tube in order to gently flush out toxic poisons, gas, accumulated faecal matter and mucus deposits, which are concurrently allowed to flow out from the colon through a second tube.

Not only does this therapy suffer from the effects of the taboo surrounding anything to do with the bowel and its function, but it also suffers because of the presumed notoriety of those who choose to use it. General consensus leads one to believe that this rather titillating group includes a certain class of male homosexual, females with eating disorders or who have an obsession with staying slim, people with more money than sense who have a mania for cleanliness and people who regularly overeat.

In recent years, in Britain, the treatment was given a torrid time by the press when it was discovered that both Diana, Princess of Wales and Sarah, Duchess of York, had had sessions with therapists known to practise colonic irrigation. However it was at this point that the tide began to turn for colonic hydrotherapy in the UK, since both women have an enormous following, and it is more than likely that their combined example has encouraged the British to be less reticent about acknowledging, and seeking help for their bowel complaints than tradition has shown them to be in the past.

In America, a more relaxed attitude to the bowel and to therapeutic approaches to cleansing it has always existed than in the UK, probably due to a mixed cultural descent, inviting and incorporating the beliefs of many civilizations, some of them still close enough to nature to follow naturopathic practices. That acknowledged, American bowel health is currently no better statistically than British bowel health, though awareness is growing faster (especially in areas such as California and in big cities) that there is a need for restorative bowel therapies such as colon hydrotherapy.

But why does anyone need such treatment in order to achieve what nature has designed with such exquisite engineering, packing the thirty-plus feet of tubing needed for successful digestion and elimination of food into a space not much bigger than a small pillow?

A glance at bowel disease statistics would seem to indicate that nature now needs some kind of help, and pretty urgently at that. If we look at American statistics, we find that an estimated 70 million people in the US suffer from bowel problems, from which 100,000 a year will lose their lives – usually from bowel cancer.

In the UK statistics reveal much the same: one in four (which is just under 15 million people) will suffer from a bowel disorder at some time in their lives, generating 10 per cent of all national health consultations.

To summarise, bowel cancer is now one of the biggest causes of death in the West. Behind those grim statistics lie the statistics of those who are 'saved' by being given colostomies –

200,000 a year in America. Further signs of malaise lead us closer and still closer to what appears to be the root of the problem: disturbances in the bowel function as indicated by laxative sales which are going through the roof – an estimated $400–600 million a year is spent on them in the US and UK figures correspond.

Orthodox bowel experts are now in agreement with the long held views of nature cure experts: that faulty diet is the focal point of the problem. The orthodox view, as expressed by the UK Imperial Cancer Fund is that 'a diet high in meat, sugar and fat and low in dietary fibre is believed to be connected'.

Speaking for the naturalists, US bowel expert Bernard Jensen, who has treated more than 300,000 people in 50 years of therapy, believes that 'poor bowel management is at the root of most health problems'. His observations led him to believe that in earlier times knowledge of the bowel was better than it is today and not only were faeces examined for parasites (world figures estimate 200 million people have parasites today) and enemas given to aid elimination where necessary, but also acknowledgment of the bowel and bowel functions was not considered taboo. He expresses the view that putting the bowel quite literally 'in the closet' is one of the worst things that has happened to health.

An interesting piece of research from Britain supports his view. In a survey conducted by the Cancer Macmillan Fund in 1988, 1,000 members of the general public were randomly questioned about their knowledge of the bowel and in particular bowel cancer. When asked which parts of the body could be affected by cancer only 10 per cent included the bowel. When specifically asked if the bowel was a place you could get cancer, only 43 per cent said yes. Commenting on these responses, leading UK bowel surgeon, John Northover, remarked, 'it (bowel cancer) is the second commonest cancer in the world and

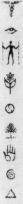

more than half the British population (on the basis of that survey) don't know about it!'

Let me be quick to say that no bowel surgeon (or possibly one in a million) believes in colonic irrigation. But let me be equally quick to say that, until a very few years ago, virtually no bowel surgeons (or possibly a few in a million) acknowledged that diet played a significant part in what was statistically seen to be an ever-increasing problem as the century advanced.

It must be taken into account that this century has witnessed epoch-making changes in our way of life due to technological inventions that have gone through a kind of sound barrier of advancement. As a result people born in this century are suffering from a time/information lag brought about by living in conditions hitherto unmapped. Will the microwave turn out to be more harmful than helpful? Will the hamburger appear in retrospect to be one of the most unhealthy dietary innovations of the century? Who knows?

What we do know is that degenerative diseases of the arteries and the colon are killing more and more people, younger and younger. And they are diseases which are largely caused by the build-up of toxic wastes in the body. These illnesses were comparatively rare in earlier days.

The arteries and colon are classic places in the body where wastes are deposited (there are 60,000 miles of arteries, 5 generously expanding feet of colon – one colon at autopsy weighed in at 40 lbs, another had a diameter of 9 inches with a passage the size of a pencil).

The main message is there for all to read: it is seen in arterial clogging (atherosclerosis), joint clogging (arthritis and rheumatism) and colon clogging (constipation, spastic colon, diverticulosis etc). Elimination and cleansing schedules are falling far behind body maintenance requirements.

Nature, due to no fault of her own, is being handed a faulty

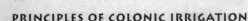

mix of fuel (food) and asked to maintain body health and integrity for our grossly speeded-up and stressed lifestyles, and furthermore to do so in an environment which requires additional elimination of toxins in order to clear the system of the products of air, water, nuclear and chemical pollution.

In the world in which our grandmothers lived we would not have needed to resort to extra efforts to clean the body's main organ of elimination – the colon – but in this day and age we need, or *may* need, every trick in the book.

Colonic irrigation does not suit everyone, nor is it appropriate for everyone, which is why this book investigates exhaustively many other successful methods for cleansing the colon of its toxic deposits derived from dietary ingested sources and from stored wastes which are now known to harbour disease, block nutritional uptake of vital minerals and ultimately promote the production of abnormal cells, as in cancer.

With the complex diseases and conditions of our time, such as candidiasis, ME, IBS (irritable bowel syndrome) – one in three are affected by this at some time in their lives – one measure is rarely enough to effect a cure. When conditions are all-embracing, their cure will need to be likewise.

As Norman Walker, another leading US bowel expert has said: 'Few people realize how directly the condition of the colon is related to weariness and part to stress and nervousness. Think how often digestive problems are worsened by family or financial problems.' Scottish bowel expert, James C. Thomson, said it in another way: 'When anything goes wrong in our lives the digestive system is the sensitive barometer.'

Overhauling the colon and cleansing it in this way involves overhauling the entire digestive system, but the bonuses are great. Reflexes on the colon reveal that it has an intimate relationship with every other part and organ of the body: so restoring

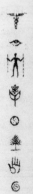

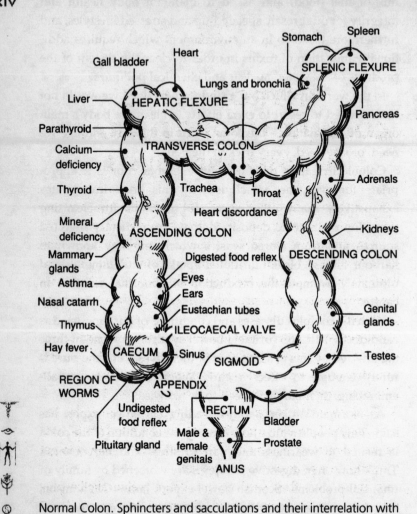

Normal Colon. Sphincters and sacculations and their interrelation with anatomical centres and pathology.

those to normal cannot but help reflect favourably on all illnesses. There is a saying: death begins in the colon: so do all cures.

PRINCIPLES OF COLONIC IRRIGATION

INTRODUCING COLONIC HYDROTHERAPY:
ITS USES AND ABUSES

For those contemplating colonic hydrotherapy, imaginations are wont to run riot as they try to visualize what the treatment will be. How do they get the water in . . . how do they get it out again . . . is there any pain? What about the terrible embarrassment if leakages or smells occur? Where does the therapist sit . . . how are you both placed? How is modesty preserved . . .?

It is perhaps a reflection of just how deep our complexes run when it comes to the bowel and its evacuation that people considering a course of colon hydrotherapy ask more questions about the procedure than about the therapy itself. However, it is usually easy to reassure them. Colonic hydrotherapy has been around for a long time. Records date back to 1500 BC and before, suggesting that by now they will have managed to get the procedure more or less water-tight.

In those days they used gourds (large melon shells) plus papyrus reeds for the piping and whatever else they could find – there is mention of the technique in older translations of the Bible. Nowadays they use a simple but effective series of sterilised tubes by which purified water, either gravity or mains-fed, enters the colon through a small tube contained in a larger, bullet-shaped, comfortably-sized speculum which is inserted into the anus and which remains there for the duration of the treatment. This also contains a separate exit tube for the removal of faecal waste. The action of the water breaks up faecal matter so that bowel contents are more easily discharged.

Those are the simple mechanics of colonic irrigation. Some have likened it to an internal bath. Possibly it would be more appropriate to liken it to an internal shower, since it is the constant flow of water into the colon which achieves the cleansing process. There is both a sluicing effect and a soaking effect, and the latter is why colonic therapy takes time: nothing should be hurried as the accumulated faecal deposits, mixed as they are with hardened colonic mucus, have usually formed into a sticky, rubbery substance which tenaciously adheres to the colon walls and needs coaxing.

Thus colonics should be undertaken as a course of treatments

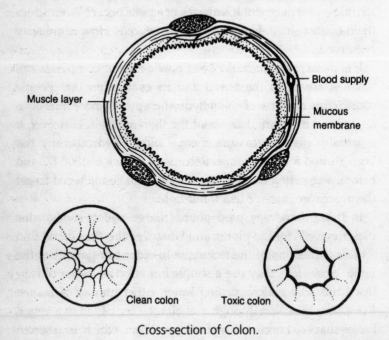

Cross-section of Colon.

(perhaps six) and initially the timing between each treatment should be such that the soaking effect of the previous treatment is not lost. What this interval represents will depend on individual health profiles.

There are full details about treatment modes and the choice of techniques (for there is great flexibility) in Chapter 2, but for now it may be more important for most readers to consider what its usefulness is in terms of bowel therapy, who it helps, what it helps, and equally importantly, who and what it doesn't help.

CONDITIONS HELPED BY COLONIC HYDROTHERAPY

Enumerating conditions helped by colonic hydrotherapy is a daunting task, since nearly every condition known to medicine will be helped by a treatment which clears the body's main sewer. Diseases are always accompanied by the production of toxins, and if these are reduced by aiding their elimination, the system struggling to fight the disease is helped in its cause. The timing of the intervention is all-important. Some people delay seeking help until challenged by serious disease: others arrive when a functional problem such as IBS affects bowel function. But by far the greatest group, experts say, are those trying to get to grips with long-term constipation.

It is not only physical diseases that are helped by this therapy but psychological ones too. Colonics can help with stress because they encourage release. When we are stressed we tend to hold on tight – and this includes the bowel contents! Releasing the bowel invites a parallel process of mental release – a true dumping process. Because of the perceived link between the mind and colon function, colonics are being used increasingly in connection with states brought on by psychological disturbances, such as eating disorders, or the addictive

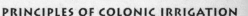

effects of long-term drinking and drug-taking, where faster and more lasting detoxification is made possible by its means. But this highly controversial and comparatively new aspect of colon hydrotherapy is not always found in the official releases of associations who control this therapy, largely because it could foster another misunderstood aspect of their already much-misunderstood work. In this context it is reassuring to know that most colon hydrotherapists have acquired extra training to help them deal with such problems.

The Colonic International Association, which has a close association with its American counterpart, the American Colon Therapy Association, lists these conditions in its official release about the treatment and what it benefits.

> constipation, diarrhoea, mucus colitis, spastic colon (often referred to as IBS – irritable bowel syndrome), diverticulitis, liver sluggishness, halitosis, headaches, flatulence, haemorrhoids, skin problems (eg acne, eczema and psoriasis), abdominal bloating, asthma, allergies, fatigue, depression and lethargy; complex conditions such as Crohn's disease[1], ME and candidiasis.

Side benefits often cite alleviation of PMT.

Included in their list is that much misunderstood section of the suffering public, clients with eating disorders such as *anorexia* and *bulimia*.[2]

Although they don't say it (to my surprise), all serious

---

[1] Not in its acute, inflammatory stage. You are advised to confer with your doctor if you have any established disease – or if you are in any doubt about the consequences to yourself. You will have to bear in mind that whatever your reason for wanting to have colonics, few doctors will approve of this treatment. They simply don't know enough about it to do so. Thus the final decision may have to rest with you; AND hopefully, another advisor who is qualified in alternative therapies, such as a naturopath or homeopath.

[2] Caution is indicated: *see Chapter 6.*

diseases are helped by colonic irrigation at some stage in their process and one disease area in particular which bears mentioning here is that of rheumatism and arthritis. These are conditions very much brought about by distortion of body chemistry, one effect of which is acidity. The clearing of the colon not only relieves the struggling system of some of its accumulated toxic load, but also the action of the water helps neutralise acidity levels.

One woman who had suffered for years with arthritis went because she was desperate and had tried everything. After a course of ten treatments she was complaining to a friend over afternoon tea that she didn't see much benefit when the friend interjected: 'Just look at what you're doing, and tell me you were doing that a few weeks ago!' Amazed, the sufferer found herself lifting the teapot and pouring tea for her friend, something she had previously been unable to accomplish due to pains in her hands.

The giving of respites in health conditions, even if only temporary (although accumulative in their effect if used regularly) has of recent years been underestimated. It helps the system to 'remember' its more normal parameters and also allows the sufferer a respite of valuable recovery time. As the alleviation of pain helps the cancer sufferer, so the alleviation of toxicity and acidity helps those suffering with joint disorders and diseases.

Another group of diseases greatly helped by this treatment is the terrifyingly prevalent group affected by various forms of arterial sclerosis, affecting either the heart, the brain or the legs. This ever-increasing degenerative disease is responsible for one in three deaths in the so-called prosperous West.

Arterial disease is a disease of clogging, where body wastes hardened by cholesterol and calcium are laid down like plaque within the walls of arteries, thus narrowing their bore and compromising the flow of vital blood to the tissues.

Cleaning the colon helps deal with the backlog, in fact it could be argued that if the colon had been able to cope with its elimination load in the first place, the condition might not have developed at all, as arterial dumping is seen as a second line of resort for the body seeking to stockpile its uneliminated wastes.

It is interesting to note that there is a very clear – and long known link – between the transverse colon and the heart and it is thought that diagnosed heart condition sufferers who experience discomfort around the navel area MAY be helped by colonic irrigation. One man, encouraged to try the treatment after his wife had been helped by it, said, 'I felt as if a stone had been lifted from my navel area. Every time I got tense I knew I got knotted up there, in the guts – I suppose that saying "knotted guts" gives the game away – knotted guts equals stress and stress equals high blood pressure for high achievers like me. Anyway, my blood pressure's dropped since the treatment and my wife tells me my temper's improved too. And unexpectedly, my sight and hearing have improved.'

It may be difficult to envisage at this stage how one therapy can claim to relieve so many diverse and, in some cases, serious conditions, which is probably another reason why colonic irrigation has such a bad name. It is indecent to claim such widespread influence on disease, reminding one rather of the successful prostitute whose client list reads like *Who's Who*.

The alleviation of so many conditions by this treatment is better understood when it is realized that any disease or condition is a sign that the body's defences have been compromised: that its elimination channels are failing to clear the body of its accumulated toxins, the effects of which then gravitate to the body's weakest point (which differs from family to family, individual to individual). This is where disease appears to start, although in fact it does not, it starts with faulty elimination.

According to an American doctor, Donald J. Mantell, who

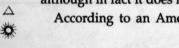

specializes in the treatment of colonic disorders, toxins from the colon can do the following:

- weaken and stress the heart

- go to the skin and cause blemishes, paleness, psoriasis, liver spots, wrinkles and other facial conditions

- go to the brain and disturb mental function and cause senility

- go to the joints and cause pain and stiffness

- go to the muscles and cause weakness and severe fatigue

- rob you of your youth, ruin your health and cause you to become old before your time.[3]

These are strong words for what is very often perceived (for a lifetime!) as the minor complaint of a sluggish elimination system. Nothing to worry about.

THE FUNCTION OF ELIMINATION: ITS VITAL ROLE IN HEALTH

When the true importance of elimination is considered, it is easier to comprehend how colonics may help a general complaint which is an ever-increasing problem in the West – auto-intoxication. Briefly, this is a condition whereby toxic wastes accumulate in certain body cells, distorting cell function and organisation in exactly the same way as alcohol interferes with the thinking processes of brain cells. However, the drinker sobers up and brain cells recover, whereas body cells such as those adjoining the

[3] From the *Nutrition and Dietary Consultant*, USA, May 1986.

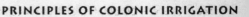

colon walls are coping with the effects of auto-intoxication all the time. Slowly, inexorably, more and more cells 'forget' their normal function and begin to go out of control. This is the kind of circumstance which can lead to cancer, where a group of cells go totally haywire and begin to invade local healthy tissue. The root cause of auto-intoxication is thought to be faulty elimination.

In our contemporary times, elimination processes are lagging behind assimilation processes, and this is now attributed to *internal* pollution caused by a faulty diet (eating food from a food chain in which chemicals are increasingly used to grow, process and basically interfere with it), plus *external* pollution (air, water, chemical, nuclear, electromagnetic) on a scale hitherto unexperienced in the history of mankind. Add to this list factors, such as the pace and stress of modern-day lifestyles, affording as they do less and less recovery time for the body, and you have a perfect formula for the destruction and degeneration of its tissues.

Technically of course, all this shouldn't be happening: body cells are in fact immortal. Cell cultures, when kept well-washed on a daily basis from the wastes produced by normal cell metabolism, have lived for decades in laboratories – one in particular lived for several decades and would technically have gone on living forever, had not human error entered the equation in the form of a laboratory technician forgetting to wash out the culture *for one day*.

Yet orthodox views hold that it is not necessary to eliminate from the colon every day! What is known is that just as carbon wastes collect in a car engine or a blast furnace, they also collect in the colon, little by little, degree by degree, until, by the time middle age has arrived, there is an ever-growing pot to prove that the colon has increased in girth by furring up. No longer do the guts occupy the space of a small cushion, but they have expanded frontwards and backwards to show the characteristic thickening known as the middle-aged spread.

It has long been ruefully acknowledged that this is an unattractive aspect of middle age, but what has been overlooked is that it is a sign of something far more serious – progressive auto-intoxication by the accumulated wastes which adhere to the colon cell walls and slowly poison them.

That this is happening when the elimination capacity of the body is truly remarkable is even more disturbing, because it suggests that all channels of elimination in the body, of which the colon is the main one but not the only one, are being compromised. (The others are the kidneys, skin, lymph, lungs, and indirectly, the liver – *see Chapter 3*).

To understand what is happening in contemporary life and why we may need additional therapies, such as colon hydrotherapy to support eliminative activities, we have to go right back to babyhood and investigate a pattern of living which in recent decades seems to have been flawed from life's start.

THE TEN-ACT DRAMA OF LIFE

Dr Erich Rauch, head of the famous European Mayr Intestinal Therapy Clinic, has said, 'Illness is a drama in 10 acts: acts 1–3 take place totally unbeknownst; acts 4–6 take place in the doctor's waiting room jammed with patients; acts 7–9 in hospital and the last act on the deathbed.'[4]

He goes on to suggest that a pattern of overeating starts in the cradle, with babies being desperately overfed. He believes that even those put to the breast, the most natural food of all, are fed too often, while bottle-fed babies are fed through teats which are too big, thus being fed both too quickly and too much.

It is very interesting to bear this contention in mind when

[4] From 'Health Through Inner Body Cleansing' HAUG INTERNATIONAL, Heidelberg, 1993.

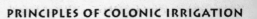

PRINCIPLES OF COLONIC IRRIGATION

observing mothers feeding their babies. One often hears exhortations such as 'a spoonful for mummy, a spoonful for daddy', while witnessing the child actually trying to avoid the proffered spoon. If we also take into account that most babies are fed milk from an animal with bones many times the size and weight of human bones, we begin to see that a pattern of overloading can be established in the cradle (where the infant learns that it can please its parents by eating what they desire), carried on through childhood (where food is given as a treat or withheld as a punishment) and ultimately suffered for in adulthood, by which time the psychological link between treat and food is so well established that it is virtually impossible to break without serious disturbance. Looking at the eating disorders anorexia and bulimia from this aspect makes them much more understandable, since they may be seen as the efforts, however distorted, of a young person attempting to try and break the conditioning of a lifetime.

This pattern becomes even more destructive to one's health when trash food is given to children as a treat (potato crisps, sweets, fizzy drinks, etc.) since that establishes poor eating preferences as well. How much better to reward a child with a special piece of fruit, or better still, with a gift or favour which has nothing to do with diet at all. If we think how often the word 'treat' comes into food advertising, it is easier to understand why so many of the population of prosperous countries are overweight – we have been conditioned to eat in response to unnatural urges.

WHERE EAST MEETS WEST: THE BEGINNING OF A FAULTY DIET

Leading London colon hydrotherapist, Margie Finchell, is an Italian, born and raised in America, who has thus experienced life in varying cultures and she has noted that amongst her more recently acquired patients are young women from the East, who arrive in London and are immediately persuaded to

change their very healthy, high-fibre Eastern diets of a little rice, plenty of vegetables and small amounts of meat or fish, to a diet rich in saturated fats and carbohydrates but which is low in fibre, and contains such things as bread, cakes and potatoes, sausages, hamburgers and so forth.

They also change their healthy habit of drinking green tea without milk to drinking tea and coffee with milk. Very soon they are constipated, overweight and spotty (the skin is one of the first places to advertise the need for colon cleansing).

As one girl said: 'I arrived there like a reed and ended up like a rush – a big fat bullrush, and I felt prickly too – inside and out. Colonic helped me get back to my starting weight but I realised that it was the slow change in my diet that had caused the problem – from fresh food to fast food; from thin, herby drinks to thick, meaty soups.'

This kind of pattern has been happening all over the world; in fact Japan, which used to have one of the lowest death rates from degenerative diseases, is increasingly moving up the scale as they adopt more and more Western eating practices.

The drama does not end there. Contemporary medical and surgical practices are aiding and abetting this degenerative process. Two such acts in the drama of illness involve the too frequent giving of antibiotics (which destroy valuable bowel flora – *see below*) and the removal (at the slightest provocation) of the tonsils and the appendix. The tonsils guard the throat and the appendix guards the colon – both provide vital lines of defence against invading germs and allogens – in fact the appendix actually secretes a germicidal fluid. To do away with these lines of defence just because they show signs of being under attack is rather like removing the radar in an airport because it might indicate an impending collision.

In Italy, the Calderoli brothers spent 30 years researching the long term effects of tonsillectomy on the system. In their book

Popoli Senza Tonsille, they formed the conclusion that not only was there a direct link between the tonsils and the colon, but also that extra strain was being placed on the colon (in particular the appendix) when the tonsils were removed. They noted too, that people who retained their tonsils had more vigour, more sex drive and were generally fitter. Ultimately the removal of any organ in the body leads to extra strain being placed on another.

Viewed in this context the removal of the gall bladder, another common operation, could be regarded as stage three in the tonsillectomy/appendectomy/cholcystectomy chain of destruction. Removal of the gall bladder leads to compromised supplies of bile, a valuable digestive aid and cholesterol controller. In fact it is a key processor of the fats so prevalent in Western diets.

Digestive processes are often further distorted by prescribed drugs, many of which affect peristalsis and cause constipation or IBS. And antibiotics, through the disruption of intestinal flora, can render the colon ripe for invasion by the opportunistic yeast candida (*see Chapter 5*). This can further undermine colon activity due to (1) toxins produced during the candida's own metabolic cycle and (2) its penetration (in its fungal form) of the colon wall, thus prejudicing that organ's ability to contain and protect the body from decomposing faecal material. When this is released continuously into the bloodstream it challenges the immune system to deal with it, thus draining that vital system's reserves. Viewed from this perspective, it becomes all too obvious how health may be compromised, item by item, gut reaction by gut reaction, over the years, until the vastly over-worked immune system breaks down, allowing one or other of the degenerative diseases to take hold – cancer, arthritis, heart disease, Alzheimer's, etc. Not a pretty picture.

Ignoring the call of nature is another bad habit often established in childhood. The very same parents who assiduously potty-train their young (often far too early and far too aggressively) suddenly forget their child's bowel now that it is under control and not a problem to them. Children should be encouraged to go to the toilet after every meal, according to leading digestive experts, who contend that if we eat three meals a day, we should evacuate our bowels as often. This, they suggest, is where the elimination backlog begins.

Consider as well the hurry syndrome of modern life (factors such as breakfast television and sitting in morning traffic jams which distract us from nature calls at the most important elimination time of day), compound this with our tendency to overeat and overdrink, and the colon is set up for trouble, as surely as if it had been programmed like a computer to deliver a given set of results.

THE ORIGINS OF UNHEALTHY EATING

Now let's look at the wider (social) pattern which is superimposing itself upon unhealthy personal patterns, such as those described above, thus causing colonic disorders to be global in their incidence.

Man was a hunter-gatherer of food until about 10,000 years ago when he began to settle down in designated areas and grow, rather than catch and collect, his food. Since that time less and less food has been eaten fresh, and more and more food which has been stored has entered the average diet.

However, this pattern did not really begin to do any harm until about 100 years ago – a time when degenerative illnesses such as coronary heart disease were still virtually unknown. In our so-called age of industrialisation, the emergent pattern began to crystallise:

- 100 years ago, only 8 per cent of our food was eaten dead.

- Fifty years ago, this figure had risen to 22 per cent.

- Now, the figure is 75 per cent and that's a conservative estimate.

Yet research has shown us that *live* food (fresh fruit, vegetables, unprocessed grains, etc) is what best sustains health. Not only does it contain energy for life, but in the case of vegetable sources it also contains fibre. Fibre, the rediscovery of recent decades, is both what keeps the colon healthy and what absorbs toxins.

BODY STORAGE PROGRAMMES AND HOW THEY AFFECT HEALTH

Besides the walls of the colon and the walls of the arteries, the body also stores its wastes in the cells of fatty tissues, thus protecting itself from the deleterious effects of its toxicity in much the same way as nuclear wastes are canned and stored in special areas. (Fat is inert – don't we all know it – and an ideal place to keep such toxins). But unfortunately in the case of the body, these areas are still re-absorbable, especially when their owner embarks on a reduction diet.

As life goes on still more places have to be found for the toxins – between the joints, in muscles, in the walls of arteries, in the colon – which is when the all too familiar symptoms of stiffness, bloatedness, shortness of breath, etc., appear. The body is running out of storage spaces. Acts 7, 8, 9 and 10 are about to begin . . . can anything be done?

Just as you can clean out a wardrobe, making more space for new additions, so can you clean out your colon. You will not achieve this overnight, any more than you achieved the accumulations overnight. But the body is remarkably quick to reward even the slightest effort. Good signs of recovery can and often do happen immediately, though in practical terms it is sensible to bargain on six months to a year, especially if there has been a faulty elimination pattern for much of your life. After that you will perceive definite signs of abatement in symptoms IF you have truly embarked on a genuine restoration programme such as those outlined in this book.

At some stage you need to find out what it is *you personally* are trying to rectify. In other words, you need to learn a bit more about your particular pattern of symptoms. For example constipation can be caused by many different factors, as can diarrhoea.

Speaking generally, both can be helped by colonic irrigation (or by other therapies described here), but the choice of supportive therapies and regimes must be made with care and caution, depending on the origins of your condition.

For this purpose Chapter 3 provides you with an insight into how your body works and a short description of the most common bowel symptoms and conditions to help you in your understanding.

It is not thought that colonic irrigation *in the hands of a qualified, well-recommended practitioner* will harm you whatever your problem, but nevertheless if you have any of the following conditions you must proceed with caution, using other, less rapid means of elimination, such as those described in Chapters 4 and 5, to help you cleanse your system.

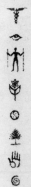

1   Malignancies of the intestinal tract – wherever they may be.

2   Any gastrointestinal disorder that makes perforation a likelihood.

3   Anal disease, such as severe haemorrhoids, strictures, fissures, etc.

4   High blood pressure. (A guideline ONLY is 160/100mmHg).

5   Severe cardiovascular disease.

6   Abdominal aneurisms and arteriosclerosis, phlebitis, thrombosis, or where there is a tendency to haemorrhage.

7   Severely debilitating diseases.

8   Severe anaemias and exopthalmic goitre.

The above list has been extracted from an excellent booklet by 'Dr Gary' (Gary N. Lewkovich, DC) who practises in California[5]. Added to these are a list from UK therapists of specific diseases and conditions, sometimes covered by the general advice above, but in the interests of being totally clear about contraindications, included again:

Diverticulitis, ulcerative colitis, Crohn's disease (in its acute, inflammatory stages), severe haemorrhoids, any colonic obstruction such as tumours or cysts in the rectum or large intestine, renal insufficiency, considerable cardio-pulmonary incompetence and megacolon. Extreme caution and medical supervision is also advised with pregnancy and anyone with a fluid retention

[5] Gary N. Lewkovich DC, 940 San Marcos Boulevard, San Marcos, Ca 92069, USA.

Those aside, colon hydrotherapy can be seen to help the majority of people with colon problems. There must be a prior consultation and careful note should be taken of case histories and symptoms: any reliable colonic practitioner will not start without this procedure.

SIGNS AND PORTENTS: WHEN TO DECIDE?

At what point – and this is the moot question – do those with colon discomfort or symptoms such as those described earlier in the chapter decide to seek help? Is this something to be done sooner or later?

The answer must lie with each individual, but here are some summarised indications:

- any established pattern, even if sporadic, of constipation (or alternate constipation and diarrhoea)

- bloating and discomfort after eating

- skin eruptions such as acne

- coated tongue, unpleasant breath, smelly wind

- anal itching (and other signs of parasites or candidiasis)

- eating disorders

- frequent headaches, with or without tiredness and lethargy including tired eyes and poor concentration/memory

- stiffness in joints, increasingly bad back

- allergy to certain foods

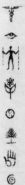

- frequent infections, especially if treated with antibiotics, including colds, 'flu, gum infections, tooth decay

- history of laxative abuse

- hormonal disruptions, (PMT, menopause, The Pill)

- two special cases, (1) after a barium meal and (2) if embarking on a therapeutic fast or dietary cleansing programme

If you decide to experiment with the treatment you are at perfect liberty to try one – or perhaps two sessions using different techniques – gravity and mains pressure (*see Chapter 2*). Some conditions/people are better suited to one technique and some to the other.

You will have on your side colon hydrotherapists, who are in the main very special people, people who may have suffered themselves and have found their own way back to health. Very often they are the people who can help with the treatment of complex conditions not fully understood or even fully-diagnosable such as candidiasis and ME. It is a requirement that therapists are nutritionally trained and many are trained herbalists as well, so can help with supportive programmes.

Colonic irrigation will not cure on its own. But it can provide the right environment, a cleansed environment, for better measures to be adopted in the future. It is not disputed that colon cleansing can be achieved by other means (*see Chapter 4*), but never so quickly, and sometimes speed is of the essence.

COLON HYDROTHERAPY:
PRACTICAL ASPECTS AND CONSIDERATIONS

The history of colonic irrigation as a therapy goes back a long way, and like most therapies of innate importance to health, records of its use are widely spread throughout the world. Thus we find accounts of it on Egyptian papyrus dating back to 1500BC, but the Chinese used it long before then. So did Ayurvedic medicine from India, where techniques such as panchakarma included colon cleansing as part of their routine.

Yogis were known to swallow lines of cloth, or, having mastered control of both the diaphragm and the longitudinal and circular colon muscles, ingested vast quantities of water (vasti) or sand (basti) through the anus for the purpose of cleansing the colon of accumulated waste.

In the early scriptures, which predated the contemporary Bible, the writings of the Essenes also describe the technique:

'Seek therefore a large trailing gourd, having a stalk the length of a man; take out its inwards and fill it with water from the river which the sun has warmed . . . hang it on the branch of a tree and kneel upon the ground . . . suffer the end of the stalk of the trailing gourd to enter your hinder parts, that the water may flow through all your bowels . . .'

It is interesting to note that in those times the exact correlation between the length of the hose and the length of the colon had already been recognised – about five feet.

Moving forwards to more modern times, we find the concept of colon cleansing persisted as an integral part of health practice until as recently as the early decades of the twentieth century, during which time attitudes to health were still being influenced by the work of such great scientists as Professor Eli

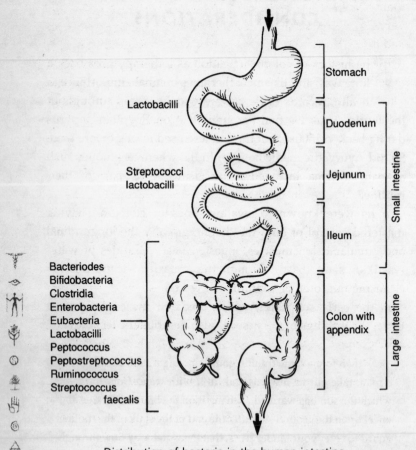

Distribution of bacteria in the human intestine.

Both pioneered research on the cause and relief of intestinal toxaemia. Both were interested in the distribution of colon flora, realising that when they were in balance they protected the entire system from the destructive effects of harmful bacteria, parasites and fungi.

Empringham actually gave rectal implants of human strains of acidophilus directly into the colon. He believed, as indeed many health professionals do today, that when taken orally very few acidophilus bacteria ever survive the digestive acids and actually reach the colon, where they are needed.

All this would seem preposterous to contemporary medical experts, as they strive to master the mystery of ever-increasing intestinal dysfunction and disease, using drugs which control colon function but do nothing to rectify its imbalances. Fashion does not always favour contemporary health it seems. In our increasingly pristine society, supporting as it does widespread advertisements for cleansing nearly everything under the sun, we have forgotten how to cleanse ourselves internally.

THE PRINCIPLES AND PROCESS OF COLONIC IRRIGATION

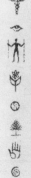

This is a technique which uses low-pressured water to irrigate the colon and cleanse it of accumulated wastes which have not been expelled due to one reason or another. Instead such wastes, by that stage usually hard and rubbery, have attached themselves to the colon walls, impairing their muscular action and interfering with the final-stage absorption of certain nutrients, additionally compromising the health of the bacterial flora in the same way that clogged irrigation channels will promote an overgrowth of weeds which choke out flowers in a garden.

The technique whereby this is done is simple, safe and

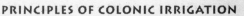

speedily effective, provided it is done by an expert. In the forties and fifties this treatment lost favour in hospitals, where it had been used traditionally to prepare patients for surgery, especially bowel surgery, and one of the reasons why this happened is thought to be because its administration was left to unqualified technicians who did not understand the few but fundamental rules needed to make the process effective. An additional factor was possibly that colonic irrigation is time and labour-intensive: giving a pill is easy. Thus purgatives and laxatives by mouth began to be used in place of colonics, regardless of the fact that the small intestine was therefore involved in the purgative process as well as the large one, thus aggravating its delicate linings and compromising its valuable function of digestion.

Unfortunately, as often happens, health custom and practice among the general public followed the example set by hospitals (egged on no doubt by commercial pressure from the drug companies) and laxatives replaced both the common use of enemas and the professional use of colon irrigation. The strength of laxative sales today indicates that constipation could be the number one condition underlying all other complaints currently afflicting the West.

As usual, this was prophesied by a few forward thinking health experts and therapists, among them America's Bernard Jensen and Norman Walker and England's James Thomson, who wrote the classic *Constipation and our Civilisation* (now released as *The Healthy Human Gut – see Bibliography*).

CONCERNS AND CONSIDERATIONS: COLON TREATMENT IN DETAIL

Anyone considering a course of colonic irrigation or hydrotherapy is understandably apprehensive about several issues: will there be discomfort or pain, will there be embarrassment, is there the slightest chance of leakage, will there be risk of infection? And – the biggest issue of all – will there be any tissue damage?

Before dealing with these, let's look at the treatment in detail. It usually starts with a case history being taken, not only about matters pertaining to the colon but to health in general. A questionnaire may be part of this introductory screening, such as that which is used by the Colonic International Association of the UK.

Because of the intimate connection between the health of the colon and nutrition, colonic therapists are usually trained to give nutritional advice as well. During a course of hydrotherapy they may want to know what you are eating, whether there are any food allergies, known or suspected, and whether there are any lifestyle problems which may be contributing to whatever symptoms there are.

The colon is a complex organ and is intimately connected to the response mechanisms of the body – response to negative emotions described before and also to positive emotions such as joy, exuberance and achievement. Success can be just as stressful in its own way as failure.

BEFORE AND AFTER

Preparation for treatment should never involve the taking of laxatives – this kind of attitude tallies with cleaning the house before the maid arrives! No therapist can judge the state of the colon if it is artificially presented. But it is wise to eat a few hours before taking a colonic in order to have something in the system to replace that which is going to be shifted. Make sure this is a meal of pure food such as fruits, grains, or vegetables, so as not to insult newly-cleansed colon walls with food containing additives, preservatives or irritants such as curry.

Expect to have wind after a colonic. Some of it will have been

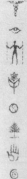

trapped in the colon and released by the treatment, the rest may have moved in to replace the faecal matter which has been evacuated. This is natural and will settle as soon as the regular digestive pattern has been re-established. (*See Chapter 4 for remedies.*)

At the onset of the treatment a gown is given to the patient to preserve modesty. The treatment itself takes about an hour, during which time water at varying temperatures will be fed into, and alternately released from the colon, together with faecal waste, at the client's pace and comfort. This exchange occurs through a closed system in which waste material is eliminated through the instrument and out via the drain line, avoiding any odour or situation which could cause embarrassment to the patient.

Do note that although some practitioners say they can do a colonic in forty minutes, any time less than an hour is not really long enough for the body to settle down and respond to the stimulus of the water. However, any more time than an hour can upset the water balance of the body, if only temporarily. It can also lead to electrolytes and other valuable nutrients being lost from the small intestine, and therapists must always watch for signs of this characteristic stage, when whitish curds begin to replace faeces.

THE PLUMBING

The mechanics of the plumbing invariably fascinate new patients, who cannot conceive of how water can enter and faeces exit through the same small tube! In fact the speculum, which is inserted into the anus and remains there throughout the treatment, contains two different tubes, one for water going in and the other for waste coming out. The need for this is obvious: water going in is sterilised and pure and must be isolated from what is coming out.

The hose which bears effluent away from the body is traditionally as long as the colon and this is for the purpose of inducing resonance. As such, it is almost like a continuation of the colon and therapists can see the contractions of peristalsis in it. Studying the pattern of these provides clues to areas of organ stress, and tapping a relevant part of the hose can induce response in a corresponding area of the colon.

Before going into the drain, the exit hose leads to a viewing tube through which the therapist observes the faeces before they reach the drain, a process which facilitates their understanding of the colon's performance and also enables them to detect any parasites or fungi which may be present.

STERILIZATION TECHNIQUES AND SAFETY

A short time ago an article appeared in the *Journal of Alternative and Complementary Medicine* about the risk of infection from colonic machines. This issue, they pointed out, is very important as viruses (including the AIDS virus) live in the lower bowel and disease can be transmitted via contaminated equipment. In Colorado, between 1978 and 1989, 36 cases of amebiasis were traced back to a colon hydrotherapy practice where insufficient care was taken between patients.

The magazine, on examining current evidence, came to the conclusion that there was no threat from modern machines which had non-return valves to prevent any waste product from contaminating water flowing into the patient, as well as which water is usually passed through an ultra-violet system which effectively kills all bacteria and viruses.

Machines such as Dotolo, Hydraline and the portable Aqua Hygiena all have such safety measures. Gravity-fed machines have a less complex construction, because the water flows

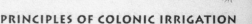

through gravity into the patient, not through a machine as such. Nevertheless it passes through a filter first, tanks are sterilized regularly and all connective equipment is sterilized between patients.

In their literature, Dotolo, who make equipment which is sold all over the world, point out that in their machines both hot and cold water filter systems remove particles as small as five microns.

All Dotolo machines use disposable speculums and hoses and they are attached to the machine through a stainless steel coupling.

THE SPECULUM: DISPOSABLE OR STERILIZABLE?

More than anything else therapists find that the lay public worry about the speculum – is it sterile, will it stay in place, will it 'leak'? Also they are concerned about sterilization of the equipment connected to them. In fact, the speculum is held in place at a distance away from the anus by the therapist and sterilization of it is achieved between each treatment by immersing it and all other detachable hoses and equipment in a powerful disinfectant (usually Virkon, which is known to kill all microbes of any kind in minutes – the recommended immersion time is ten minutes). However, most therapists now prefer to use disposable speculums and tubes so that each patient receives a new, individually-packaged, completely sterilized object, the seals of which are broken in front of the patient.

Those who do not use disposables and who prefer metal speculums for, they say, very good reasons, (more 'solid', with a protective 'collar' to prevent over-insertion, more comfortable, less likely to contain little 'scags' of plastic) are absolutely meticulous in their sterilization procedures, either using an autoclave

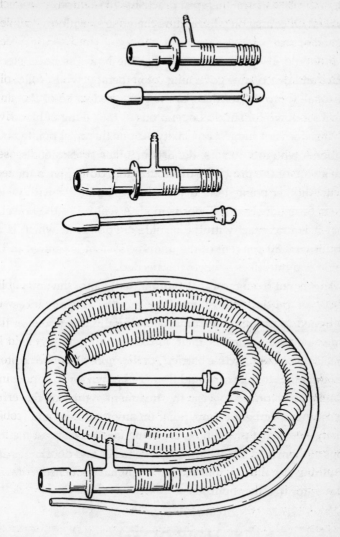

Top: Stainless steel speculums, with insertion parts. These slide into speculums for entry purposes; are then removed to allow water access and waste excess pipes to be attached.
Bottom: Disposable speculum with anal sigmoid safety insertion shield (to protect and control degree of entry of speculum).

PRINCIPLES OF COLONIC IRRIGATION

or, in the case of one therapist practising in London, a pressure-cooker! Of course they have more than one speculum, usually a dozen or so.

It should also be understood that the bowel is not a sterile place and procedures governing colon therapy, whilst following hospital-approved routines, are not required to be of the standard set down for surgical operations or the taking of blood.

This does not suggest any laxity. As one therapist pointed out: patients who are doctors, dentists or other professionals, who are aware of the principles of sterilization, don't give a thought to it. Another pointed out that the knives and forks with which we eat are not sterilized, nor is food. A feature of the bowel is that it is in contact with the outside environment which is no doubt why 80 per cent of the immune system is centred in the colon and intestines – where it is needed.

This is not to suggest that putting things into the anus is the same as putting things into the mouth. Gastric juices are designed to put an end to many potentially dangerous organisms ingested, whereas their introduction through the anus meets no such protective barrier. All the more reason for colonic irrigationists to take care, and they are known for it. A potential patient may prefer to visit the treatment rooms of the colon hydrotherapist before embarking on any treatment and see for themselves what precautions are being taken. The most meticulous of them actually disinfect light switches and doorknobs and anything else the previous patient might have touched. All wear gloves for treatment purposes.

HOW OFTEN, HOW MANY AND HOW MUCH?

Frequency of treatments is as difficult to answer as the proverbial 'how long is a piece of string?' Each person differs in both their needs and responses: however, it is usual to embark on a course of six to eight treatments to begin with, and wise to have the first two or three close together. 'Vulcanized' bowel contents will take time and soaking to shift and it may take several soakings to start the process off. If treatments are close together the colon does not have time to revert to its former state.

Will there be pain? The treatment is remarkably free of any real discomfort though some abdominal cramps are to be expected when evacuating strongly, which happens from time to time. These are no different from what is felt when evacuating the bowel under normal circumstances, in fact they are more gentle. Sometimes the influence of the water can cause gurglings – as can the presence of trapped gas. This is transient. One has to remember that the colon therapist has sat through many sessions and has 'seen it all before'.

WATER

Amazingly, the amount of filtered water used can be as much as 15 gallons – under extreme circumstances this figure can double but this is unusual. The temperature of the water is varied during the session in order to relax and stimulate the bowel alternately.

Water pressure is another issue of great importance. Colon machines have control devices which cut this down to two pounds per square inch (2psi). But Milo Siewart, a trainer of colonic therapists in England, points out that in the course of a treatment water pressure is prone to rise to equal that in the mains (general water supply) pressure – another reason why timing is so important. Thus a colon therapist may well ask a patient if they are 'feeling the pressure' or a similar question to monitor the true state of affairs as the session proceeds. It is important to say what is being felt at any given time during a

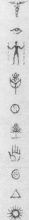

colonic and never to put up with discomfort beyond an acceptable level (which differs from patient to patient).

GRAVITY V. MAINS-FED MACHINES

There are two types of equipment used for the giving of colonics – gravity-fed equipment and equipment which is plumbed into the mains where the water is conducted through a machine especially designed for this purpose. There are strong advocates for both: gravity is considered the gentler and more natural treatment: machines are more technical and more sophisticated. Adjuncts to the basic therapy can be given with machines, such as the administration of oxygen.

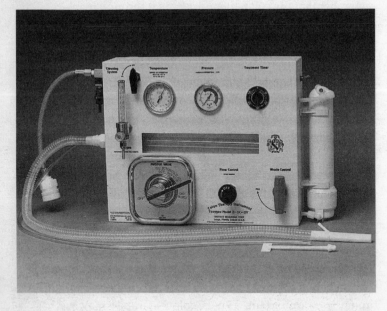

This is a portable machine for colonic irrigation designed and built by Jonathon Bailey of the International Colon Hydrotherapy Foundation (see Useful Addresses). It is equipped to provide ozone therapy as well as hydrotherapy for the colon.

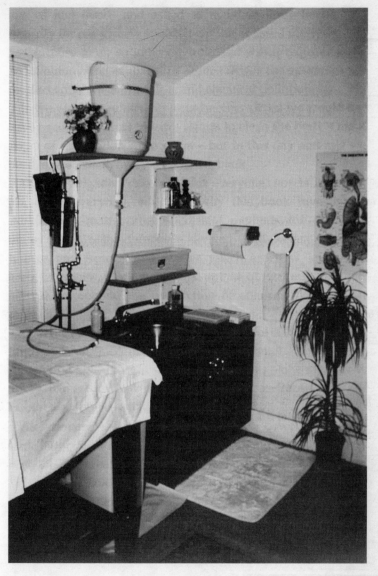

Gravity-fed colonic equipment in the Devon-based therapy rooms of Roger Groos. Water tank (on top shelf) is about three feet above patient.

The potential patient is advised to try both and see which suits better: there is no doubt the treatment differs. Some believe that problem bowels respond to the more subtle effects which can be induced through gravity-fed machines: therapists using mains-fed machines would defend this position strongly. As in all forms of personal therapy, it is invariably true to say that the skill of the therapist matters more than the type of equipment used.

BEFORE LEAVING

At the end of the treatment a patient needs time to recover and to eliminate any final material not yet evacuated. It is important to wait until comfort is restored before venturing forth and not to rush this process. After this point has been reached some therapists give an implant of acidophilus to reseed the colon; technically to replace flora which may have been lost during the washing out process. The efficacy of this will depend both on the quality of the flora given in the implant (which should be of human origin) and whether the bowel is ready to accept it.

Many colon experts prefer to encourage natural restoration of bowel flora by supportive dietary measures, such as the taking of whey, and foods rich in lactic acid, such as natural yoghurts and sauerkraut and juice 'musts'. These are discussed in Chapter 4.

There is a widespread belief that having colonics washes out the good flora and as such does as much harm as good. Actually the treatment, in clearing the walls in which the good flora embed themselves, promotes the production of healthy flora rather than compromises it.

Abdominal massage is often performed during the process of the therapy, since this greatly facilitates both release and comfort. Sometimes this takes a more specific form, in that reflexes in the colon relate to every organ of the body, and if there is disturbance in an organ it can be treated immediately by massaging the relevant reflex area of the colon. One therapist recalls doing this for a woman suffering from breast cancer. As she massaged this reflex area, the woman experienced a hot rush of extremely sludgy material from the bowel. Hot rushes of this kind are not uncommon and are thought to be associated with release of toxic 'hot' material from the colon walls and crevasses.

Sometimes external castor oil packs for the abdomen are advised as these also facilitate the elimination of waste. This treatment was often advocated by Edgar Cayce and can be extremely soothing. The best time to apply such packs is the night before a colonic and the method is as follows: pour 4oz of caster oil into a bowl and soak an old, clean flannel cloth in it. Prepare a heating pad or hot water bottle. Place a sheet of plastic (a dustbin bag will do) on the bed and cover it with a towel. Lie on this and place the oil-soaked flannel cloth on your abdomen. Cover this with another sheet of plastic and tuck it around your waist. Add another towel. Finally place the heating pad over all this and leave on for one to one and a half hours. The effect is both soothing and stimulatory.

An interesting study from Korea[1], in which 85 people suffering from various forms of constipation were monitored whilst being given a course of colonics, mentions that stomach

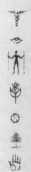

[1] *Clinical Research for Faeces* Medical Treatment Dept., Taejon University Hospital, Seoul, Korea October 1986.

packs were often used during that study and consisted of hot soya bean paste – which is also known to draw out toxins.

STUDYING THE EVIDENCE

The observation of faeces is an integral part of the diagnostic aspect of the treatment, and patients are thereafter encouraged to observe their faeces at home as once something is known about them they provide valuable guidelines to what is needed and not needed in the diet.

Not only size, but shape and colour can tell you how well your bowel is working and alert you to any significant changes. Size and shape indicate speed of transit through the gut and this is of key importance in judging how active and responsive the colon is. One British gastroenterologist has devised the Bristol Stool Form Scale which divides stools into seven distinct types, progressing from (1) extremely constipated to (7) diarrhoea. (It is interesting to observe that whilst colonics are more frequently given for constipation and for sluggish, spastic bowels, the opposite condition of diarrhoea does not necessarily preclude its sufferers from needing the treatment. Faeces may be 'hurrying past' the cause of irritation on the colon walls, just as they may be 'lingering' in cases of constipation.)

Type 1   Hard lumps like nuts.

Type 2   Lumpy sausage.

Type 3   Sausage with cracked surface.

Type 4   Sausage with smooth surface.

Type 5   Soft blobs with well-defined margins.

Type 6   Fluffy with ragged edges.

Stools also vary in colour and changes in colour are significant.

Pale faeces, like oatmeal, often follow a bout of diarrhoea. The less bile there is in faeces, the lighter they are, so this can also indicate blockage in the bile duct or deficiency in producing bile. Bile is a vital digestive aid and without it certain foods are not fully digested. A diet very high in fat can sometimes produce pale stools, as can failure to absorb nutrients in the small intestine. Observation of conditions like these can be invaluable aids to securing appropriate treatments.

Bright red blood in the stool is most often caused by bleeding haemorrhoids, but can occasionally indicate bleeding due to disease in the colon and this sign should never be neglected.

Dark faeces are usually the result of dietary factors, such as taking an iron supplement or drinking beetroot juice, red wine or eating dark foods such as spinach.

Black faeces may indicate occult blood, ie bleeding higher up in the digestive tract. This, like overt blood, must never be ignored. Jet black, tarry stools are caused by an actively bleeding stomach ulcer.

Ideally a healthy stool should float in the pan. However taking bran will produce this effect artificially, therefore floating does not invariably indicate a healthy, self-sufficient colon. Discontinue the bran for three days and see if the stools still float.

ACID/ALKALI BALANCE

This is measured by taking the pH of the colon contents. Water, which has a neutral pH, is 7. Anything above that is alkaline, anything below is acid. Contemporary observations of the pH of colons have led specialists to believe that the normal colon is

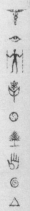

alkaline but this is because of the widespread nature of faulty diets rich in meat and other putrefactive material. In fact the healthy colon is slightly acidic, which is exactly the environment favoured by the acid-loving (hence their name) acidophilus.

When the colon is alkaline the protective bacteria do not flourish and this encourages the growth of opportunistic flora such as candida. In fact modern colons are characteristically imbalanced, which may account for the prevalence of colon conditions, such as IBS, today. A leaflet from the Dotolo Institute of America, which involves itself not only in the making of colonic machines but in research, informs us that every year 140,000 Americans are diagnosed as having colon-rectal cancer, of which 44 per cent will die of the disease. This is often the end result of conditions such as colitis and ileitis, from which, the Institute say, at least two million Americans suffer, 100,000 of whom will, in consequence, be forced to have a colostomy. These conditions are a direct result of neglecting such symptoms as constipation, diarrhoea, IBS, etc.

In fairness, sometimes people seek help from their doctors for their bowel problems only to find the side effects of the 'cure' almost as bad as the complaint, so they abandon their quest. Modern medical therapy for the colon is largely directed towards controlling symptoms and rarely gets to the seat of the problem – although more, at last, is being understood about the

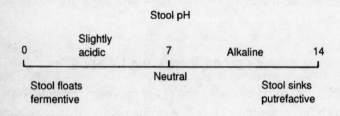

Healthy colon flora are indicated by slightly acidic stool which float in the pan.

OXYGEN, THE NEW ADDITION

Of recent years, colon therapists have started to use a variety of adjuncts to basic colon therapy and one of the most controversial of these is oxygen.[2] Essential for life, oxygen is taken up less and less readily as we age, live in polluted areas with oxygen depletion, or simply fail to breathe deeply enough. There is no doubt that oxygen introduced into the colon does find its way immediately into the bloodstream and as such must both purify and enliven colon wall cells.

In *Healing Within*, written and published by Stanley Weinberger (*See Bibliography*) a long-time US colon therapist and health authority working in the San Francisco area, oxygen therapy is described thus:

> 'There is no comparison in the way one feels after a cleansing with the new procedure with oxygen . . . Some authorities state that, litre per litre, more oxygen is absorbed though colon cleansing than through the lungs. This not only helps to heal the affected tissues in the colon, but also allows the oxygen to pass quickly into the bloodstream and bathe all the cells in the body . . . Colon therapy with oxygen has an antihelmintic action, that is, parasites are removed . . .'

There are those who contend that the flora of the gut are anaerobic and as such should not be introduced to oxygen. As yet the

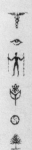

[2] Information about oxygen therapy in its many applications can be had (with SAE) from Derek Wolfe, 'Newton Mill', Newton-St Petrock, Nr Holdsworthy, Devon EX22 7LP.

38 treatment has shown only benefits. Again, it is an option to be decided upon between patient and therapist.

HERBAL TREATMENT AND SKIN BRUSHING

Two more common adjuncts to a course of colon therapy are to introduce herbs to the colon during the therapy and to employ the supportive technique of skin-brushing while the course lasts.

Herbs are usually introduced during the treatment by means of diverting the main water flowing into the bowel to allow the absorption of the contents of a bottle holding the liquid infusion of herbs. These may be soothing, as with camomile, or have various effects according to the condition being treated. Typical examples of herbs used in this way (or by oral infusion) are fennel, goldenseal, acacia gum, yellow dock root, plantain, blessed thistle, cloves, red clover, cornsilk, butternut bark – obviously the choice requires an expert knowledge of herbs.

Substances may also be given to stimulate the bowel – sometimes coffee is used for this purpose: rectally introduced coffee has a long history of use in stimulating the liver and bowel to release its toxins (NB: It should always be organically grown coffee.)

Kombucha[3] is a naturally fermented drink made from tea, the taking of which in the East has long been associated with longevity. When the tea fungus works it actually produces oxygen making this an extremely natural way of working with this element.

Skin brushing also has a long history of use in detoxifying programmes. Skin is one of the five main organs of elimination, and brushing its surface with a firm body brush, preferably of

[3] See Useful addresses.

natural bristles, helps remove both dead cells and toxins attached to them.

Start with the feet and work upwards towards the heart with long smooth strokes, then brush up each arm towards the heart, up the lower body, across the shoulders and down from the head. Be gentle on delicate skin areas, such as breasts and face. Five minutes daily is sufficient to leave skin glowing. Continue with this until the course of colon therapy is over. (If you skin-brush all the time, your body gets used to it and the cleansing effect wanes. Do it for a few months, then stop for a few months. Then begin again).

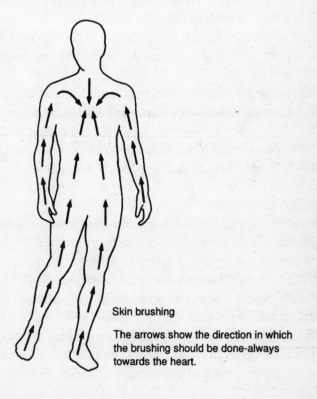

Skin brushing

The arrows show the direction in which the brushing should be done-always towards the heart.

Examining the tongue will give a good indication of how your cleansing is progressing. The towel-like surface of the small intestine, with its enormous surface area, is not unlike the surface of the tongue. In *The Healthy Human Gut* (*see Bibliography*) C. Leslie Thomson summarizes the various appearances of the tongue and what they can tell about health conditions:

Geographical Tongue: Thomson says this resembles the surface of a map, with some parts red and raw, and others heavily coated with whitish catarrhal material. This is said to indicate long-term (now septic) constipation where putrefactive wastes are being reabsorbed into the system.

Broad, pallid, thick tongue (frequently bitten because too big for the mouth): indicates an excessive carbohydrate intake – starchy and possibly sugary too.

Small red tongue : acidity which may indicate irritated stomach walls, or nervous tensions of a deep and lasting kind.

Ulcerated tongue: tiny sore spots, painful, out of proportion to size and colour – may indicate disturbed blood conditions. Can be due to local irritations such as a broken tooth or smoking.

Large 'piecrust' tongue: pale and puffy showing teeth indentations. Fluid retention.

Adjuncts such as this to basic colon hydrotherapy, whether diagnostic or treatment-based, can be helpful in arriving at an exact understanding of the source of a health problem, but it should always be remembered that the treatment works regardless of diagnosis or help from other sources. It is almost embarrassing when confronted with a therapy which helps nearly every complaint known, especially when very few actual studies have been done and most of the positive evidence has come from the combined experiences of those who have the treatment and those who give it. Since the treatment itself is or has been under a cloud, so are the opinions of patients and practitioners involved in it.

There are some exceptions to this rule: several studies *have* clearly shown an association with constipation and slow transit times of foods through the colon and breast cancer. And one Korean Study showed a very positive result from treating constipated patients with colonic irrigation. After a course of colonic irrigation 56 per cent were considered cured. (It should be noted that traditional colon therapy there incorporates, like most holistic therapies, the use of supportive measures such as oxygen and herbs.)

Putting two and two together, it can be seen from just these two studies that (a) health can be negatively affected by having sluggish bowels and, (b) sluggish bowels can be positively affected by having colonic irrigation.

WHO IS HELPED?
BENEFITS AND APPLICATIONS

Although few, if any, claims are made by practitioners, many have cancer patients[4] on their books and many cancer patients are helped by the treatment, because cancer is a disease brought on by toxicity. Similarly arthritis patients are helped considerably. Arthritis, characterized by tumour-like growths in joint spaces, is recognized by some experts as having similarities to cancer. It is known that in these cases the enzyme system needed for digesting and breaking down tumour cells has become defective, as has the immune system. Since both of these activities are largely centred in the colon and small intestine and digestive organs, it surely makes sense to begin healing in those sites.

[4] Not intestinal cancer.

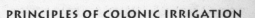

The association with heart conditions and unhealthy colons is also well-established – again, some experts liken the build-up of cellular and fatty deposits in arteries with uncontrolled tumour-growth activity.

ALCOHOL AND DRUG WITHDRAWAL AND FOOD SENSITIVITIES

Some of the lesser-known uses of colon hydrotherapy relate to drug withdrawal and in fact to any addiction/withdrawal programme, because the treatment speeds and facilitates detoxification. If the substance causing addiction is still in the system, obviously it is going to be harder to give up. There is real value in this aspect of colon hydrotherapy, as the therapeutic mode is psychologically supportive as well as detoxifying.

ANOREXIA AND BULIMIA: A SPECIAL CASE

Using colonics to control weight is an extremely vexed area of colon therapy, especially if an underlying psychological condition exists. The tyranny of slenderness, one of the most destructive fashions of our times, is discussed in Chapter 6.

THE BEAUTY ASPECT

Health and beauty are inextricably linked: restoring the one guarantees improvement in the other. Eyes clear, skin improves in colour, spots disappear, hair texture improves. Besides these visual benefits, people note that their level of alertness improves.

Mood is also very affected by the bowel, and studies of the elderly, who sometimes suffer from atonic constipation (due to loss of muscle tone extending to the colon muscle which is involved in peristalsis) indicate that having a colonic invariably cheers them up. This effect is not exclusive to the elderly: in fact the observation of it has prompted well-known health therapist and author Jan de Vries to express concern about people becoming addicted to the treatment because it makes them feel so good afterwards. Almost anything in life can be abused, it seems, even a treatment for controlling abuse!

CRITICISMS

Evidence does not seem to support the view that regular colonics do any harm IF those 'overdoing' it do not suffer from any contra-indicating complaint. Dogs given enemas every day for five months in a row showed remarkably few changes in bowel mucosa or flora – which puts in question yet another well-aired criticism of colonic irrigation – that it compromises bowel flora. However, any cleanse will result in some surface flora being removed and these should be replaced (by anal implant or by mouth).

If taking by mouth, stomach-acid proof supplements (such as DDS-1, *see Useful Addresses*) are advised and should be favoured. At the very least a potent live acidophilus cultured from human strains or made fresh from cabbage – see Chapter 4 – should be taken in substantial quantities (*see also Chapter 5 and Useful Addresses*).

PUTTING POWER BACK INTO PERISTALSIS

Of obvious use in atonic constipation, and with any complaint in which bowel muscle tone is weak, eg spastic colon, colon hydrotherapy is invaluable for all conditions of constipation, as

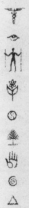

well as for chronic wind, or gas problems. It is also to be recommended in both the preparation for and alleviation of the colon from substances used for medical tests, such as those involving the taking of barium meals, or other dyes and substances.

WATER BALANCE AND BODY SALTS

There is little, if any, evidence to suggest that the electrolyte and fluid imbalances sometimes observed after colonics in people with serious system malfunctions/conditions, such as megacolon, neurogenic constipation, cord lesion, or advanced malignancy apply to the average person.

Obviously, since the colon's function is to absorb water under normal circumstances, there will be an increased amount to deal with under abnormal circumstances, such as colon irrigation, but only temporary disturbances in the levels of some body salts have been observed and these are neither long nor at levels which could be considered significant. An excellent study was completed by several research scientists at the College of Naturopathic Medicine in Florida[5] on the effects of colon hydrotherapy on serum electrolytes and they came to the conclusion that 'with ambulatory patients who were free of serious pathology . . . no patients experienced any clinically significant complications or complaints during or after the course of treatment'.

Obviously this water-absorbing factor is why extreme care must be taken in treating anyone with fluid level imbalances, whether brought about by high blood pressure, heart failure, kidney malfunction or by the toxic conditions of faulty metabolism. In fact, in the normal person the diuretic activity of the body

[5] Paper available from Dotolo Institute, address in Useful Addresses (with adequate return postage).

is increased by colonic irrigation: just as electric storage batteries last longer by being encouraged to fluctuate from fully charged to fully discharged, so the human system functions better when it is challenged to express the full range of its natural responses.

NEUROTIC NEEDS: USE OR ABUSE OF COLON THERAPY?

There is a certain type of person who is obsessed with cleanliness and this is often associated with bowel disorders, prompting the sufferer to seek what they see as help in 'getting clean'. Most colon practitioners are well aware of the signs of such complexes, but within reason, may seek to help the person by giving some treatment. Practically every colon therapist says that the therapy goes far beyond the mechanics of clearing the bowel and seems to encourage release on all levels. Sometimes the deepest fears can be expressed and helped during this release promoting therapy.

However there are therapists practising in the alternative health field who believe that care must be taken to discourage those who are using the treatment to satisfy neurotic needs or slimming goals. Jan de Vries cites one young woman who took a year to recover under his care from excessive use of colonics. One swallow does not a summer make, but nonetheless this aspect of criticism would seem to be directed to the need to invigilate and educate colonic therapists into awareness of the responsibility to their professional reputation. There are greedy doctors, greedy dentists – avaricious professionals in every area of health. Vigilance on the part of professional controlling organizations and on the part of prospective clients is the only protection against this universal phenomenon.

On the other side of the coin, an amazing number of people scorn what they suspect to be the 'pain or pleasure' aspect of

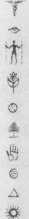

having colon therapy. One leading London colon surgeon said, disapprovingly, he 'was sure people got pleasure out of it', as if pleasure was an unacceptable facet of healing. Case history memoirs of therapists who have been giving the treatment for years (*see Chapter 7*) suggest this aspect is more prevalent in the minds of the beholders than in the beholden (the patients) and that when it does occur it is harmless.

ADJUNCTS AND HOME SUBSTITUTES TO COLON HYDROTHERAPY

Cleansing of the colon is considered to consist of a four-fold option programme involving: 1 colonic irrigation; 2 enemas; 3 fasting; and 4 herbs in whatever combination seems to be appropriate.

All of these will be discussed in the course of the book but in this chapter about functional techniques it is appropriate to look at the option of enemas.

ENEMAS

This process (for some) presents a horrifying prospect which has no doubt been 'coloured' by the memories of older members of the family who may have recalled being given enemas in childhood by a stern and relentless parent seeking to treat a variety of conditions from parasites (worms) to constipation.

Enemas form an integral part of some healing therapies, such as the Gerson therapy for cancer, which prefers this technique to full-scale colon hydrotherapy, possibly because it is less invasive for those who are seriously ill and who may also have cancer lesions or complications in the colon.

Basically the technique differs from hydrotherapy in that (a) it only treats the final section of the bowel – the rectum, and possibly part of the descending colon; (b) water is retained for some time during an enema whereas in hydrotherapy there is a constant flow in and out, and (c) other substances besides water are likely to be used, though not necessarily.

BENEFITS

Those who use enemas say they can alleviate symptoms such as headaches, nausea, the cramps of food poisoning, overeating, constipation, diarrhoea, bloatedness, in a very short time. Clearing the rectum encourages the contents of the colon to move and stimulates peristalsis, thus helping with the elimination of toxins.

ENEMAS: SELF-ADMINISTRATION

Enemas can be self-administered using an adult ear syringe or an enema bag (available from larger chemists) using techniques such as the following:

Prepare one pint of water at 80°F (just under the temperature of blood). (If an enema bag is used, one-quart of water is needed). USE ONLY PURIFIED OR DISTILLED WATER.

Squeeze the air out of the syringe or bag and take up the liquid, to capacity, eliminating as much air as possible. Place a small amount of sterile lubricant on the tip of the syringe and around the anus. Lie in a prone position on your back, bending your legs at the knees. Slide a cushion covered with plastic, then towelling, under your hips to raise them slightly. Gently and slowly insert the tip into the rectum, approaching from between, not around, the legs so as to push the tip in straight. Keep in this position until the liquid is absorbed (you may have to fill the syringe several times, so keep the container close by. Never overfill to discomfort or distension.)

Roll over onto the right side for a minute to give the solution every chance of entering the ascending colon and even reaching the caecum (unlikely). Hold the liquid for as long as comfortable,

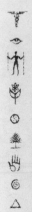

then eliminate on the toilet. Repeat several times if necessary.

Implants can also be given this way, using less water (so it can be retained, not expelled) into which acidophilus has been dissolved. Some therapists also recommend the use of powdered whey solutions. There is an excellent account of this in David Webster's little book *Acidophilus and Colon Health*, distributed by Nutri-Books, PO Box 579, Denver, Co 80217, USA. It is also available from specialist bookshops and health stores in the UK. Make sure that every single thing used when administering this treatment (including your hands) is made and kept as clean and pure as possible.

During a fast (*see Chapter 4*) daily enemas for up to seven days can help with the discharge of toxins but there is, as with all bowel treatments, the caveat to be extremely gentle. Bowel specialists warn that there is a small, but finite risk that if you put tubes into the bowel you can damage the delicate wall. However, with care, lubrication and a careful approach this need not happen. Dogs given daily enemas over a five-month period showed only slight skin changes as a result of the frequent entry of enema tips.

CAVEATS

- Never do this or any other bowel treatment to excess.
- Always discuss with a qualified therapist what you are planning to do and for how long.
- Buy your products from reputable suppliers.
- If suffering from haemorrhoids, do not consider this self-applied technique until the haemorrhoids are under control (*see Chapter 4*).
- Try to learn a bit about how your colon and digestive system work so that you can understand better what your system needs (*see Chapter 3*).

PRINCIPLES OF COLONIC IRRIGATION

UNDERSTANDING THE COLON AND DIGESTION:
ITS FUNCTIONS AND MALFUNCTIONS

I t has been said that the English prefer to think of the colon as a mark of punctuation! However, they are ultimately forced to acknowledge its alternative meaning when symptoms begin to impinge upon their consciousness, such as indigestion, intestinal discomfort, haemorrhoids and constipation, by which time the bowel problems are usually well-established, and probably have been going on since childhood.

This head-in-the-sand attitude can never be good for colon health, nor can the faults be remedied until the entire digestive system is better-understood as an entity. When that happens light dawns, causes of discomfort can be tracked down, and subsequent care of the colon, of the entire digestive system, becomes a straightforward business, because it makes sense.

THE DIGESTIVE PROCESS

The *Encyclopaedia Britannica*, in describing the digestive system, has this dry comment to make: 'The digestive tract begins at the lips and ends at the anus.' It is very necessary to acknowledge the implications of this when practising colon care. What goes through the lips inevitably ends up in the colon, which is no

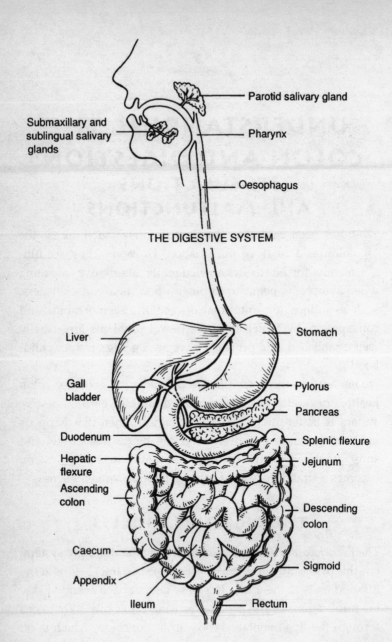

THE DIGESTIVE SYSTEM

Parotid salivary gland

Submaxillary and sublingual salivary glands

Pharynx

Oesophagus

Liver

Stomach

Gall bladder

Pylorus

Pancreas

Duodenum

Splenic flexure

Hepatic flexure

Jejunum

Ascending colon

Descending colon

Caecum

Sigmoid

Appendix

Ileum

Rectum

stainless steel tube, although as dietary habits go, it seems that
many people regard it as one.

Stainless steel tube it may not be, but nonetheless in health the colon (and indeed the entire digestive tract) should be regarded as separate from the body, a continuum of the external environment. Obviously, at some stage of the digestive process, the nourishing contents are transferred across to the body through what is effectively the semi-permeable membrane of the intestinal walls, but this is what the limit of the transference should be in *ideal* health, thus isolating any potentially dangerous microbes and pollutants that may get into the gut from the external environment.

What happens, though, is often very different, giving rise to an internal pollution which is just as serious as that of our external environment. The microcosm reflects the macrocosm.

The process of digestion really starts in the mouth when the enzymatic digestive juices in saliva mix with food (how well depends on how well it is chewed). Food then proceeds to the stomach, where strongly acidic gastric juices attack it to break it down further and render it digestible – and in the process, if said juices are acid enough, kill any invasive bacteria which may have contaminated the food. (Imagine how much good the taking of antacids does for this de-infecting process.)

After several hours in the stomach (depending on the type and combination of food eaten) the contents, by now nearly liquid, begin their journey through the intestines, starting with the small intestine. There, more digestive juices and enzymes are contributed by the liver and pancreas to aid digestion further.

The intestines are an amazing 25 feet long – that's longer than most people's gardens – and when their function is considered the inference may well be that they *are* the garden of the body, containing as they do intestinal flora (microbes, fungi, bacteria) which help break down food just as the microbes in a compost mixture aid the transference of nutrients to the soil.

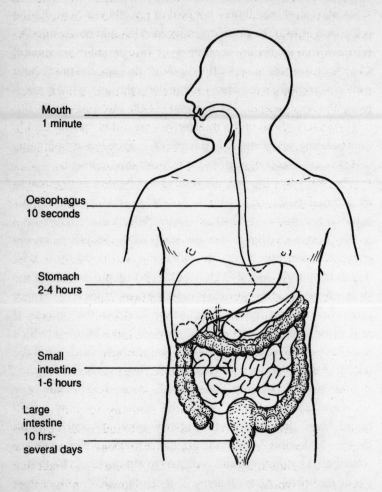

Mouth
1 minute

Oesophagus
10 seconds

Stomach
2-4 hours

Small
intestine
1-6 hours

Large
intestine
10 hrs-
several days

The Digestive System. The diagram illustrates the average time that food spends in each part of the digestive system.

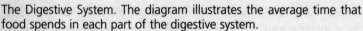

Whereas food remains in the stomach for only 2–5 hours, it will remain in the small intestine for as long as 10, because this is where the chief process of digestion takes place. In fact, until not very long ago, it was believed that the only purpose for the following large intestine (the colon) was to store condensed food residues left over from the small intestine's efforts until they were eliminated as faeces. Now it is known that the colon completes the process of digestion in more ways than one.

In his book *Stomach and Bowel Disorders* (*see Bibliography*) Jan de Vries describes the colon as being 'designed to expedite waste matter from the body and is also involved in absorption of nutrients from food'. Modern research further indicates that the healthy colon produces its own energy as well – through the short-chain fatty acids formed there. If this is so the phrase 'to have guts' becomes all the more meaningful, implying a sort of strength derived from the bowel when all is well with digestion.

This is better understood if we think of the reverse – the depleted, drained feeling which comes from indigestion (think of Christmas lunch). Experts also tell us that bowel energy is affected by the length of time food stays in the gut: the longer, the less energy. In this respect vegetarians win out over meat eaters: the average transit time for them from eating to elimination is 18–30 hours, whereas the average for a meat eater is 60.

While food remains in the gut it is decaying and decomposing and therefore giving off toxins, so to reduce this process as much as possible would seem sensible. Does this mean the whole world should become vegetarian? There is no doubt that colon health would be improved by it. However, meat eaters can have healthy bowels IF they also eat plenty of fibre and IF their diet contains foods that will preserve the health of intestinal flora (*see Chapter 4*).

THE IMPORTANCE OF BOWEL FLORA

There are no less than 2–4lbs of flora (parasites) present in the bowel of the average human gut, some of them potentially lethal if allowed to escape into the bloodstream. Candidiasis, caused by the overgrowth of one of them, candida albicans, is a classic example of what can go wrong if their respective balances are not preserved. Just as weeds can take over the garden, choking out desired plants, so can opportunistic bacteria and fungi overrun the bowel.

Only the healthy environment of an intact intestinal wall can keep such monsters at bay as E. coli, salmonella, streptococci, poliovirus, pseudomonas, trichomonas, entamoeba, bacteroides, clostridium and candida. These dangerous bacteria are kept in check mainly by the beneficial bacteria (chiefly bifido bacteria and lactobacilli). These help to control viruses, fungi, yeasts and even worms which try to inhabit the gut.

It is chastening to realize that these disease-causing bacteria are present in the human gut all the time and are only kept in check by the delicate balance of the intestinal flora and the action of the immune system of the colon. Thus if infection does break out in the body it usually reflects unhealthy intestines. The first line of defence has failed us.

Viewed in this light, it can be seen that trying to control such outbreaks with antibiotics may seem to work but is not really getting to the root of the problem; furthermore, it is now widely known that antibiotics kill not only the bad bugs but the good ones, including beneficial bowel flora such as acidophilus, thus setting up a potential chain reaction in the decline of bowel protection.

This is just the sort of pattern of events which people who suffer from bowel disorders often describe: first infection and treatment with antibiotics, then bowel symptoms such as wind,

griping, etc. all of which worsen with time under the influence
of stress or subsequent infections.

BOWEL FLORA: A DELICATE BALANCE

Intestinal flora inhabit the mucus which lines the towel-like
intestinal walls, which forms an ideal substrate for them while
it is healthy: unfortunately, dietary factors and poor elimination
tend to render mucus sticky instead of slippery, hard and
rubbery instead of soft and pliable. This sticky mucus then
adheres to bowel wastes, leaving deposits which encourage
infection, putrefaction and degeneration of intestinal tissue.

Every gardener knows that only weeds will grow on clogged
soil. So it is with the bowel: the healthy flora get overgrown by
the opportunistic bacteria and the results lead to a variety of
symptoms ranging from 'minor' ones of bloating, smelly wind,
bad breath, indigestion, constipation, right through to conditions involving the whole body, such as allergy, toxicity or
frequent infections. Furthermore, the build-up of mucus and
waste means that food moving through the colon makes less
and less contact with colon walls, therefore its nutrients are
absorbed less.

In the long term we may develop one of the increasingly
common colon infections or diseases such as candidiasis (yeast,
thrush), colitis, IBS or diverticulitis.

The longer food remains in the colon, and the less effectively
it is transported out, the more likely are conditions to arise such
as those described above. This is why fibre and fluid are two
highly important and vital factors to colon health: the one
brushes the walls of the colon and the other lubricates and facilitates exit of faeces. These are discussed in Chapter 4.

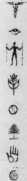

COLON ANATOMY

The colon itself is a complex and peripatetic organ which begins on the right side of the body, just above the right hip bone, rises to cross the stomach at about navel level, then descends down the left side of the body until, with a significant kink or two (a bit like the U-bend of a sink and just as potentially clogging) it turns towards the centre of the body and becomes the rectum, the last part of the bowel before evacuation. (NB: The skin lining the rectum is much the same as the delicate skin lining the mouth – which is surely the greatest incentive of all to 'clean up the act of defecation' and speed up its process, especially as it is known that long-term insults to the skin of the bowel predispose it to cancer.)

AS TIME GOES BY

Whereas the small intestine is only 1.2–1.6 inches in diameter, the colon is approximately 2.5 inches wide, but its length is only one fifth of that of the small intestine, i.e. about 5 feet long. However, the nature of the colon walls, built to accommodate varying volumes of faeces, means that they can expand to occupy an enormous amount of space, ballooning backwards, forwards and sideways, and eventually crowding out their 'flat-mates' (the uterus, vagina, ovaries, prostate, bladder, kidneys, etc) until those organs 'feel the pinch' and start malfunctioning too.

Furthermore, the colon can become misshapen, becoming pinched in places, bagged in others. The famous US bowel surgeon, John Harvey Kellogg, who during his lifetime is said to have performed over 22,000 bowel operations, said he'd never seen a completely normal colon. When the colon becomes constricted in some places and expanded in others, peristalsis

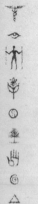

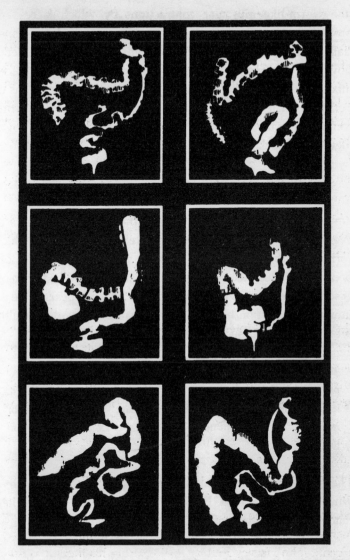

The above 6 pictures of prolapsed, distorted, twisted, sickly-looking colons are exact reproductions of X-ray negatives of the colons of apparently healthy . . . people.

Colon Health by Dr N. W. Walker/ Publisher: Norwalk Press/Prescott Arizona.

PRINCIPLES OF COLONIC IRRIGATION

58 (the worm-like muscular contractions by which faeces are propelled along the intestines) becomes disturbed too, especially if there are kinks in the colon which prevent its contents flowing. The increasing bulk of encrusted mucus/faeces mixture on the colon walls also slows down the contractions of peristalsis. The result is usually chronic constipation, a word coming from the Latin *constipatus* meaning 'to press, or crowd together, to pack or cram'.

THE COLON AND REFLEXES

We also know that within the colon there are reflex points to every part of the body. Just as there are areas on the feet which correspond to every organ in the body, so are there on the colon. Because of its connection to every organ in the body, the colon is sometimes used as a diagnostic tool. There appears to be an intimate connection between colon health and cardiac health, prompting experts such as Dr W. Bezley to say:

> 'there are few phases of cardiac trouble in which disorder of some part of the alimentary tract is not causatively associated – in fact it may be that almost every chronic disease known is directly or indirectly due to the influence of bacterial poisons absorbed from the intestines.'

These poisons gravitate to weakened spots in the body, areas where there may have been a previous injury, an inherited tendency, or a pattern of childhood illness.

THE IMMUNE SYSTEM AND THE COLON

It is thought that as much as 80 per cent of immune response is activated from the colon. Certainly it is well-supplied with lymph material in its walls (as indeed is the small intestine through groups of lymph cells called Peyer's patches), also there is a plentiful supply of enzymes in both the colon and the small intestine and these are the immune system's first line of defence.

The appendix too, is part of the colon's immune defence system – its safety valve for isolating infection. To remove this without good cause may not eradicate the infection, but simply drive it deeper.

Obviously, an immune response working from a clogged location will suffer in its effectiveness and looking back it seems incredible that what was known and recognized in 1912, (when a group of 57 leading British surgeons met to discuss the importance of bowel hygiene and the increasing problem of auto-intoxication of the colon), has been so easily forgotten. At that meeting, at the Royal Society of Medicine, they identified twenty-two poisons as originating from the toxic colon:

phenol, cadaverin, agamatine, indol, sulphuretted hydrogen, cresol, butyric acid, botulin, putrescin, urobilin, histidine, ammonia, muscarine, methymercaptan, indican, methygardanine, indoethylamine, sulpherrglobine, ptorrmarropine, pentamethylendiamine, neurin and sepsin.

In America, bowel experts, such as Bernard Jensen and Norman Walker, were familiar with a test for one of these poisons, indican, which was regularly done to check the auto-intoxication level from the bowel where it was suspected: now that test is no longer generally available.

The decline and fall in bowel care on both sides of the Atlantic and indeed throughout all of the Western world can be directly associated with the rise of degenerative disease. When the immune system of the bowel becomes compromised extra

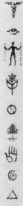

work is forced on the remaining systems of elimination, the liver, lungs, kidneys, lymph gland and skin. This is why symptoms sometimes reveal themselves in secondary sites, such as skin eruptions, bad breath, liver spots etc.

SUFFERING IN SILENCE

It is difficult to conceive how we can suffer such progressive destruction in the bowel and not realize it. The reasons are thought to be two-fold: firstly the bowel is poorly-supplied with nerves which convey pain, and secondly, with continued abuse of any body system, reactions which indicate disharmony become suppressed. Thus the bowel of a baby quickly reacts to unfriendly substances, but as time goes by primary reactions transpose themselves into secondary ones such as allergies, just as these in time will transpose themselves into more serious conditions and ultimately into disease.

STRESS AND THE BOWEL

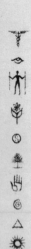

There is another factor operating in the bowel which does absolutely no service to normal bowel function and that is stress. Peristalsis is quickly arrested by stress. This is a throwback to our ancestors, who were hunter-gatherers. When faced with danger, defecation often occurred immediately (this is a response everybody has known) in order to relieve and lighten the person and ready them for combat: after that peristalsis was arrested because ingesting and digesting food was not on the agenda until the crisis passed.

We are left today with the inheritance of a bowel which responds in this way, yet our lifestyles have moved on: crises today are rarely matters of life or death yet the bowel responds to them as if they are. While on the one hand, bowel nerves do not convey pain, they do convey stress. In fact, the entire digestive system is one of the first areas to respond to disturbances to the equilibrium.

This whole issue of stress and its complex and diverse effects on the bowel and finding precise ways of handling it is presented in Chapter 6. Suffice it to say that nervous reactions may be responsible for many functional bowel disorders, such as IBS, constipation, diarrhoea, etc, and some may be so deep-seated, arising in babyhood or childhood, as to be totally inappropriate for the contemporary picture of life.

Thus it is often a *combination* of factors, including bad dietary and elimination habits, plus the vital element of stress, that conspires to defeat healthy colon function. Fear, anger, grief, anxiety, all affect the digestive system in different ways: the trick is to discover which one is the active ingredient in our own personal lives and find therapies to relieve it.

VALVES AND FLEXURES: POTENTIAL SITES FOR PARASITES

There are two locations in the colon which are particularly predisposed to problems; the ileocecal valve leading to the caecum, and the sigmoid flexure. The first is situated in the hollow of the right hip bone and marks the junction between the small intestine and the colon.

Not only does stress affect the opening and closing of the valve, but it also affects the caecum itself, which, being sac-like, is prone to harbour bowel contents when peristalsis is arrested, which then decompose and form an ideal breeding ground for parasites.

No one today can believe themselves to be exempt from the threat of parasites, which are estimated to affect 200 million of the world's population. Quite apart from the undesirability of

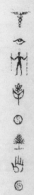

62

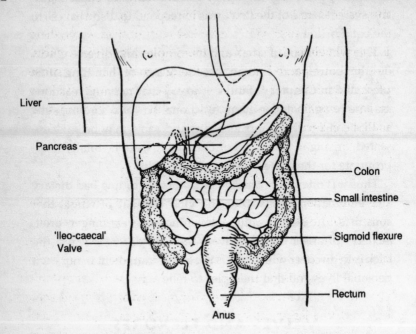

Liver

Pancreas

Colon

Small intestine

'Ileo-caecal' Valve

Sigmoid flexure

Rectum

Anus

The 'ileo-caecal' valve and sigmoid flexure form two sensitive areas of colon anatomy in which flow can be impeded.

harbouring parasites (one in four are said to have round-worms – *see Chapter 5*) they sap nutrients and body energy. In fact more people die of parasite infections, diagnosed and undiagnosed, than of bowel cancer, the incidence of which is second only to lung cancer in men and breast cancer in women.

The sigmoid flexure on the other side of the body is also prone to infection. It represents the sharp down turn made by the descending colon as it transforms into the rectum, the final organ of elimination. This sharp bend, like the U-bend of a sink, is terribly prone to clog up. In his book, *Tissue Cleansing Through Bowel Management*, Bernard Jensen describes how as many as

may be held up in this crook waiting to be evacuated.

Since by this stage faeces have lost most of their water, there is every likelihood of sticky residues adhering in the crevices. This pressure-packed situation is thought to be the classic cause of diverticulosis (a condition where the bowel wall weakens under the strain and balloons into sacs in which decomposing material collects).

THE MUCUS FACTOR

Obviously the bowel needs to be lubricated to facilitate the moving of its contents, and cells in its walls produce copious supplies of slippery mucus for this purpose. However, the nature of Western diets predisposes the formation of yet more mucus of a viscous nature, especially in response to eating dairy products (milk, cheese, yoghurt, cream, ice cream, fromage frais etc), and to a lesser extent meat, fish and eggs. Soya products are also mucoid-forming, so protein intake should always be balanced by a plentiful supply of fresh fruits and green vegetables. Sticky mucus hardens on bowel walls and impedes peristalsis.

The mucus factor seems to be one of the key problem areas of bowel function. When excess mucus is produced as a reaction to an irritant in the bowel (whether food, drugs or whatever) it backs up into other mucus-producing channels of the body, such as the sinuses and the lungs, causing symptoms which seem to be unrelated to the bowel.

Many children are allergic to milk, many more to wheat, but the resulting mucus surfeit is more often detected from asthma or hay fever symptoms or from frequent colds than from the initial site of the problem, the colon. To worsen the picture, drugs are given to treat these secondary symptoms, which will

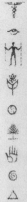

probably further exacerbate mucus production in the colon! No illness can ever be arrested until its true origin is discovered: the following Rakes's progress shows what can happen if it is *not* discovered.

FROM CONSTIPATION TO CANCER IN A LIFETIME OF EASY STAGES

Scaremongering is only justified if all the signs point to its being both accurate and constructive. There seems little reason to doubt the words of nearly every bowel expert, whether orthodox or alternative, concerning the health-destructive habits of diets rich in refined foods (such as sugar, white flour and both artificial and animal fats) and poor in fibre, and their deleterious effects on the bowel.

Here is what the eminent British bowel surgeon, John Northover, has to say: 'The high prevalence of the disease (cancer) is associated with environmental factors, diet-related.' He goes on to cite two main dietary factors: absence of fibre and high amounts of animal fat and protein. Together with Joel D. Kettner, Assistant Professor for Sciences, Surgery and Community Medicine at the University of Manitoba in Canada, he has written a book, *Bowel Cancer: The Facts* (Oxford University Press, 1992) in which highly convincing evidence is presented about the progressive decline in bowel health which has occurred in Western civilized countries.

The authors build up a highly convincing picture of substantive evidence which suggests that diseases of the bowel are proportionately connected with the degree of departure of any society from the type of food eaten by man in his wild state, ie when he was a hunter-gatherer.

They quote information gathered from Africa by Dennis

Burkitt, an English surgeon who worked there (Africans traditionally eat diets high in vegetable fibre and low in refined foods of any kind – their food is also mostly eaten fresh) who published what has become a classic paper on the epidemiology of cancer of the colon and rectum. 'Based on his own studies as well as those of others, Burkitt concluded that diet was the main cause of bowel cancer (and several other conditions of the bowel such as piles and diverticular disease, as well as other diseases like diabetes and varicose veins).'

This understanding helps us to help our children, but in the meantime there are many people well on the road to life who need to know how the pattern of bowel disease develops down the years so that intervention can be achieved at the point appropriate for them so that bowel (and indeed general) health can be restored.

FUNCTIONAL AND ORGANIC: A MATTER OF DEGREE

The medical profession divides bowel problems into two main categories: functional, meaning something is wrong with the way the bowel works; and organic, meaning something is wrong with the parts (ie organs). Obviously, the latter is more serious than the former, since the latter represents established disease.

What they don't often say is that the difference between the two is only a matter of time. Logically, if something is not working well then it puts strain on other working parts and may have widespread repercussions.

Imagine bowel disorders and diseases as a rather negative tree, probably growing in swampland. (Swamp has all sorts of connotations with excessive or bottled-up emotions, as well as with an unhealthy environment, which seems perfectly appro-

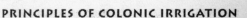

66   priate.) Such a tree could be said to have been rooted in one's past and an upbringing which inadvertently incorporated all the prevailing misconceptions about health, dating right back to babyhood and stern potty training (implying to the infant the need to hold back the bowel) through factors, such as convenience foods, sedentary lifestyles and a fair degree of stress – environmental, emotional, economic – the possibilities vary with each person. Along comes the first of the bifurcations in the tree: functional complaints such as constipation (very common), indigestion (ditto), diarrhoea (branching in the opposite direction to constipation) and a variety of secondary branches, such as food (or other) allergies (eg asthma and hay fever) other skin rashes, sinus trouble, or frequent infections.

When puberty arrives, hormonal problems can enter the scene – every girl knows how notorious the pre-menstrual phase is for affecting bowel function – usually causing constipation. Pregnancy and dyspepsia seem inextricably linked: the menopause leads to other complications. For men, unevacuated faeces can affect sexual and ultimately prostate function. And for both sexes the wearing of tightly-belted clothing encourages another ill, such as shallow breathing. Factors such as irregular mealtimes, rushed lifestyles, the taking of specific drugs and medications, like alcohol, aspirin, the pill, tranquillizers, antacids, antidepressants, iron pills, high blood pressure tablets, street drugs, coffee, tea, not forgetting smoking, also play their parts, most having either stimulatory or suppressive effects on the digestive system. And obviously if something is taken or done on a regular basis then its effect will be both constant and progressive.

Enter what is usually the chronic constipation and indigestion stage, where the taking of indigestion tablets and/or laxatives seems the only everyday solution to normalize bowel and digestive function.

Wrong. This may well be the critical point at which the foliage of an established bowel dysfunction begins to form. Dr John Northover explains what can happen if, for example, laxatives are taken regularly (in my introduction I quoted the figure of $400–$600 million a year for the USA and in the UK estimates vary from £20–£50 million. Consider also the sales of Tagamet, for indigestion, thought to be one of the record bestselling drugs of all time).

'Regular use of any pharmacological material is something to be avoided if possible . . . stimulatory laxatives such as those containing senna can, over a long period of time change the nerves to the bowel and actually *increase* constipation. One very obvious abnormality you sometimes see is the colour of the lining of the bowel changing with those who have used laxatives over many years. It is called "melanosis" a pigmentation which can in a way be likened to skin damage.'

The opposite problem, diarrhoea, may be caused by irritants in the diet (past or present) or by overstimulation of the bowel nerves, either through emotional causes or metabolic ones (body chemistry). Diarrhoea usually responds to similar dietary and stress-control approaches as given for constipation – the two seem to be opposite sides of the same coin. However, specific details of such approaches will obviously vary.

Conditions such as the following could be considered to represent what MAY become the intermediary stages between functional disorders and bowel disease.

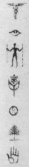

1 Adhesions from any 'ectomy'.

2 Ballooning and its opposite, constricture (including diverticula). Also hernias.

3 Mucosal dysfunction.

PRINCIPLES OF COLONIC IRRIGATION

4   IBS and colitis.

5   Any condition which affects bowel nerves or function, such as back injuries, prolapses and emotionally-based eating disorders such as anorexia or bulimia.

6   Fissures and haemorrhoids.

7   Atonicity (usually senile in nature).

8   Liver and gall bladder problems.

9   Parasites and candida.

10 Long-term artificial treatment of chronic constipation and diarrhoea.

11 Addictions of any kind.

12 Food allergies.

13 Malabsorption syndromes (as in pernicious anaemia, coeliac disease etc).

All or any of these conditions may just as easily lead to health as to disease. There is a saying: 'the secret of good health is to have a serious condition and cure it', the implication being that in so doing you learn how to look after yourself. Hence the following 'flowering' need never happen.

DISEASE: THE FINAL STAGE
BUT NOT THE FINAL CURTAIN

Even established bowel diseases will respond to determined and dedicated treatment. But 'treatment' is a word which has come to imply either surgery or some other form of orthodox intervention, such as the use of prescribed drugs, chemotherapy, etc.

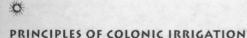

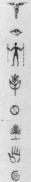

Before embarking on such a course it is wise to consider the very rich and real alternative treatments now offered in bowel care. Sometimes these may be embarked upon as real alternatives, and other times as complementary treatments to those required by the disease and its stage of development.

At the disease stage, medical advice and supervision is to be expected, but this does not prevent the patient from learning as much as possible about their condition, either through reading books (preferably not just reading literature given out in doctors' surgeries which will most probably present only the orthodox view), or by contacting organisations representing those who have had the disease.

Since the final choice/veto rests with the individual, it seems wise to consider all options. However, the alternative field of health can represent a bewildering and unfamiliar field to members of the general public who often have no idea of their disease or treatments for it until it is diagnosed. Thus consulting an alternative health professional (possibly a well-known author or contributor to health magazines or a diversely qualified health professional) such as in the fields of nutrition and/or naturopathy, should balance the viewpoints.

When disease strikes, many people tend to regard themselves either as patients or, worse, as a statistic: they look fearfully at the death rates, weigh up their chances and very often give in.

Cancer is NOT a death sentence. I personally have an old friend who had bowel cancer many years ago: so do most people you care to speak to. That said, the following diseases must never be taken lightly, and any successful treatment must involve not just treating the part that's gone wrong but overhauling the WHOLE system. And – what must make eminent sense especially in respect to bowel diseases – cleansing the system. How can treatment begin otherwise?

BOWEL DISEASE: A SYNOPSIS

The main diseases of the bowel are as follows:

1   Polyps and benign growths

2   Diverticulitis

3   Ulcerative colitis

4   Crohn's disease

5   Cancer of the colon and rectum.

Polyps and benign growths can usually be cured by surgery, the sooner the better as they are known to develop into cancer over time.

Diverticulitis is a condition characterized by the development of small pouches in the wall of the bowel. They are directly derived from the greatly increased pressure required to force hard stools along the bowel – and are hence the result of constipation. If faeces become trapped in the pouches infection can cause inflammation and abdominal pain, usually in the left lower abdomen. (Jan de Vries graphically calls the condition left-sided 'appendicitis').

Ulcerative colitis and *Crohn's disease* are both inflammatory diseases causing pain, diarrhoea and weight loss. They are both thought to be connected with abnormal immune response, possibly due to an earlier infection. For example, there is speculation that a divergent strain of the measles virus may be implicated in Crohn's disease.

Treatment for these type of diseases must then be aimed at strengthening immune function, for which an all-embracing health programme must be entered upon. Programmes (or advice on where to find help in selecting them) are offered for

The ultimate, most dreaded bowel disease is of course cancer, and the fact that it strikes the colon much more often than any other part of the digestive system suggests that it is a question of contact with decomposing, unhealthy faeces. It is interesting to note that studies of cultures such as the Mormons and of primitive cultures whose diets mostly come from vegetable sources, indicate that such people are relatively protected, not just from cancer but from most forms of bowel disease. So it seems that meat and animal fats are the culprits, together with low fibre foods.

SYMPTOMS TO CONSIDER

Lastly, here is a list of symptoms which must never be overlooked:

1   Chronic or persistent pain and/or tenderness.

2   Chronic indigestion, diarrhoea, constipation.

3   Alternating diarrhoea and constipation.

4   Swelling and distension of the stomach.

5   Wanting to move the bowels and being unable to.

6   Pale, ill-formed stools.

7   Blood in stools, including occult blood which may darken their colour.

8   Unexplained weight loss.

OTHER CONDITIONS AND DISEASES OF THE DIGESTIVE SYSTEM

Conditions such as hiatus hernias, or diseases such as stomach or duodenal ulcers or coeliac disease (caused by allergy to gluten) are not really the subject of this book, although many of the treatments and measures suggested in it (apart from colonic irrigation which must never be attempted where there is ulceration or inflammation unless specifically ordered by a doctor) may prove helpful.

It is generally accepted that colonic irrigation is not appropriate for cancer either, and yet there have been cases, not necessarily of colon cancer, where colon therapy has helped immensely to detoxify a system struggling against cancer. One of the major problems confronting those trying to get to grips with this disease, a problem fully recognized by avante-garde experts, such as Dr Max Gerson, is that as cancer cells die as a result of constructive therapy, their toxins are released into the system. These must be dispersed if the patient is to recover. However, such decisions must be made on individual cases with full medical consultation, preferably from an expert trained in modern approaches to cancer.

THE COLON: AN OVERVIEW

Jason Winters has said in his book, *In Search of the Perfect Cleanse* (*see Bibliography*):

'The colon is dark, damp and warm – the perfect place for the breeding of germs and unfriendly bacteria. It is said that it is impossible to ever gain perfect health without cleaning the colon.

The time has come to recognize its importance, to take it out of the closet and give it the attention it deserves.'

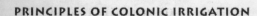

PRINCIPLES OF COLONIC IRRIGATION

WORKING
TOWARDS WELLNESS

Dramatic effects can be experienced after the first colon cleansing programme: the worse the state of the colon, the more dramatic the effects tend to be. Eyes clear, skin colour and texture improves, odd complaints disappear and there is a general feeling of well-being and levity. But this state of affairs will not last unless a concerted effort is made to maintain the progress achieved.

This requires knowledge: of both what to avoid in the future and what to favour. It is no longer possible to leave all health decisions to health experts, whatever their designation. This is your body, your house for this life and you have to know how to spring clean it and keep it sweet and healthy. Householders who assiduously clean out their refrigerators and food stores on a daily or weekly basis, throwing out all produce that has passed its best, have to start thinking like this about their body. And where there has been an accumulation of waste produce of many years' duration, as with the colon, a programme has to be instigated whereby stored wastes are systematically cleared, a bit at a time, so as not to clog the elimination systems, until true homeostasis has been reached.

And once that plateau has been reached that too has to be maintained by a revised, more biologically friendly, life pattern.

Staying well should be thought of as an ongoing process which lasts a lifetime, until we really are ready to move on.

STEPS TO RECOVERY

Let's assume that your colon-cleansing urges have been stimulated by a course of colonic irrigation – or if you cannot or do not favour this treatment, you are ready to begin with alternatives. What is the programme?

The functioning colon needs:

1   sufficient water

2   good nerve tone

3   good muscle tone

4   adequate circulation

5   the right biochemical nutrients

6   the right food intake.

This may seem obvious but already changes will have to be made in many lifestyles.

Liquid intake will have to be reviewed, as will vitamin B intake, which supports nerve function. Sufficient exercise will have to be undertaken to promote good muscle tone and improve circulation. As for the right biochemical nutrients and food intake – that could revolutionize the entire diet!

FIRST THINGS FIRST

There is a clear order of priorities when embarking on any health cure and the order for the colon is:

1   Clear the toxins

2   Acidify the colon

3   Promote or implant beneficial colon flora.

This may seem a bewildering programme for the average person who may not know how or where to start but it's really very simple if taken stage by stage. But it may be reassuring to know that ANY positive effort on ANY level, however sporadic and however out of sequence, will ultimately benefit the health of the colon and hence general health. So if some steps simply can't be contemplated at any given time, that is no reason to avoid implementing others.

DIAGNOSING YOUR PROBLEM

Earlier in the book I gave a list of conditions which may contribute to colon dysfunction. Recapitulating here for the purpose of self-diagnosis, these conditions are as follows:

A diet too rich in animal and processed foods; too low in vegetables, fruit and other natural foods; the regular taking of any specific medication for whatever reason (eg the pill, steroids, antidepressants, laxatives, tranquillizers, antibiotics, even aspirin on a regular basis or some vitamins – especially high-protein formulas and most iron pills; depressants such as alcohol, stimulants such as cigarettes, tea or coffee; the over favouring of some foods (monotony in the diet) which may cause sensitivities, hidden or unknown; the taking of street drugs and glue sniffing; food/drink excesses leading to vomiting or diarrhoea; drinking chlorinated/fluorinated water; emotional stress; inability to express feelings; hyper-ventilating or chest breathing; inhibiting clothing; bad posture or back/nerve injuries; unsuspected radiation and other forms of pollution, especially chemical pollution

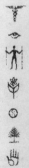

from additives or household/garden products; and air pollution (especially in cities).

After selecting which of the above may apply to your particular problem, you will be more clear about which sections of the ensuing therapies and measures may improve your condition. Later in this chapter there is also some brief advice for natural ways of controlling known bowel conditions and diseases.

DIETARY AIDS AND MEASURES

One of the surest ways to correct and control bowel dysfunction is through diet. Basically this means avoiding some foods and favouring others. Unfortunately, this may initially seem like avoiding most of the foods you love, whereas what it really means is avoiding them until you have learned how to substitute them with foods which taste the same as they did but are made in different ways and of different ingredients. This may mean buying a few recipe books which teach you how to select and prepare 'safe' foods and devoting a few weekends to shopping for them and/or preparing them for later consumption.

WHY ORGANIC?

Does this mean organic? Ideally yes, but everyone knows how difficult this can be to locate and how expensive it is. This is changing as demand for such foods grows, but meanwhile the careful selection of fresh foods and the careful washing off of any surface sprays with Milton's solution or even scrubbing with a natural bristle vegetable brush may be an acceptable intermediary stage. However, try to locate, as soon as possible, your nearest source of organic produce. Many of the larger chains of supermarkets now stock organic lines. Gather together signatures and request that they are stocked in your area. Demand them and they will be supplied – eventually.

It is not just that organic produce is free of traces of agricultural chemicals but also that it is completely different in composition. Organic produce is grown on healthy soil; the emphasis being on soil health not plant health. Thus the plants take up from the soil what they naturally need. In the case of produce grown with the aid of artificial fertilizers, the soil may or may not be healthy and it may or may not contain vital trace elements (for example selenium is widely deficient in British soils).

Inorganic plants are artificially fed or forced, so you get the equivalent of human oedema (water retention) underlying what is likely to be a sodium/potassium imbalance within their tissues. This imperfect mineral balance is then passed on to the consumer who is already likely to be eating food containing far too much salt and too little potassium, since current Western diets favour salty things, such as crisps, sausages and other prepared savouries. Of course, the produce looks wonderful: it is plump with water and succulent, whereas organic produce can be a bit stringy and tough. But it is not natural and very probably not wholesome, in the true meaning of that word.

That, in a nutshell, is why organic foods can and must return to foodshelves. Inbred, overcultivated foods are simply not as lively nor as hardy. When we eat fresh food we eat not only substance but lifeforce. That is the vital electrical component of life, the energy whereby cells organize and reproduce themselves. Photographs which show the life force emanating from plants clearly indicate that it is far stronger in organic produce.

FOODS TO FAVOUR; FOODS TO AVOID

Foods to select for healthy eating may vary in minor ways from person to person but essentially the basic rules apply to all:

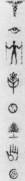

1   Eat as much fresh food as you can, ie fruits and vegetables. Vegetables, if cooked, should be as lightly cooked as possible, either stir-fried or steamed. Favour fruits and vegetables in season as these are what the body needs at that time. The more brightly the foods are coloured, the better, since highly coloured foods tend to contain more of some vital nutrients such as beta-carotene.

2   Drink as little tea and coffee as possible and work towards the idea of cutting them out almost completely. Not only are they addictive and are therefore affecting the entire system, but both contain substances which do not agree with the colon. Try a selection of herb teas until you find some which you like. Particularly good (for health) are camomile, comfrey, bancha, pau d'arco or lapacho and peppermint.

3   Give up tap water altogether (chlorine suppresses acidophilus bacteria). Favour still *mineral* water over carbonated as the latter affects the acid/alkali balance of the body besides causing gas. NB: Learn the difference between mineral water and spring water – one (the former) is stringently monitored and controlled, the other is not.

NEVER drink large quantities of any liquid with food and NEVER drink iced water at that time as this slows down the enzyme activity needed for digestion. Anything drunk too hot is not good either – digestion functions best at body temperature.

4   Try to eat less wheat-based foods and cows' milk-based foods. This means bread, cakes, biscuits, some pastas, savoury snacks, as well as all dairy products, including milk, cream, fromage frais, and commercial yoghurt (a *little* butter is acceptable). The reason for cutting down on these

PRINCIPLES OF COLONIC IRRIGATION

two food categories is that Western diets contain too much 79 of them and eating too much of any one type of food tends to produce not only dietary imbalances but also food sensitivities. They also tend to increase acidity.

FOOD SENSITIVITIES; KNOWN AND UNKNOWN

Sensitivities occur when the immune system begins to respond to a food, usually frequently ingested, as if it were a poison, a foreign substance. Such false alarm activities can so exhaust the immune system that it is left with no reserves necessary for fighting real microbes or controlling the production of rogue (faulty) cells which may become cancerous.

This sensitized reaction (which can be perceived as bloating, wheezing, fluid retention, flushing, palpitations, headaches or anxiety) is partly caused by long-term ingesting of a surfeit of a particular substance and partly caused by the presence of foreign substances in such foods in the first place; usually because they have been artificially bred, selected and grown.

Species of wheat from which bread, etc, is made today have been selected not because they are hardy and would survive in nature but because they produce a grain with qualities desired by millers and manufacturers of bread products. The same applies to milk-producing cattle, who for simple economics are often fed with artificial foods (sometimes derived from excrement!) plus regular supplements of antibiotics and hormones (a) to prevent infections which would lower profit margins and, (b) to promote tender flesh and/or milk production. Traces of all of these things appear in the end product, and may be recognized by the immune system in the gut as toxins and unwanted substances.

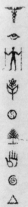

PRINCIPLES OF COLONIC IRRIGATION

Regrettably, the same is true of all but organic poultry and eggs (of which only four a week should be eaten).

There are other (inherited) reasons for food sensitivities and it is wise to have suspected (or indeed unsuspected) sensitivities checked, especially if allergic reactions are experienced anywhere in the body. This can be done very simply today by a blood test, thereby eliminating the lengthy procedure of eliminating suspected foods one by one. It can also be done by kineseology (muscle-testing) or dowsing (*see Useful Addresses*).

In place of wheat, try to substitute breads and produce made with oats, rye or rice. In place of dairy products based on cow's milk try to eat foods made with goats' or sheeps' milk. There are, however, two cow-based cheeses which are 'more acceptable' than most – Swiss cheese (such as Gruyere, Emmenthal) and cottage cheese.

5   Eat less red meat and try to get protein from vegetable sources such as legumes, grains and pulses. Brown rice is a wonderful food, with its protein and carbohydrate content perfectly balanced for human consumption. Because the grains are unpolished they contain fibre as well.

Instead of meat, favour fish (especially deep sea fish) and organically produced chicken and game. Game and lamb are two sources of protein which can be eaten in moderation as the animals get their food from nature and thus it is less likely to contain substances which the immune system finds foreign.

Try and avoid pork altogether. Many societies have placed a ban on eating pork and there are very sound reasons for this. It is simply not a pure meat.

6   Cut fat consumption to a minimum, especially animal fats. These clog the system besides introducing into it toxins stored by the animal in its fatty cells. Use cold-pressed olive

oil which not only reduces cholesterol levels but also aids the colon in its functions.

7 Take care with citrus fruits, especially if you suffer from a tendency to acidity or if rheumatism runs in your family.

8 Try to get some bitter and sour tasting foods into your diet as well as the sweet and salty ones. Sour and bitter tastes stimulate enzyme production such as bile, which is an invaluable aid to digestion and absorption.

Here is a list of the foods most often found on the dietary blacklist for one reason or another: margarine (because of the chemicals and heat used in processing); animal fats; saturated oils; salt; sugar; vinegar; fermented foods and pickles; foods containing fungi and moulds such as mushrooms and blue cheese; monosodium glutamate; processed foods such as luncheon meats; pork and beef; starches; white flour and products made from it; soft drinks; beer and spirits (try to drink only organic or good-quality wine); chocolate; tea and coffee; and too many rich nuts such as Brazils or macadamias, and all peanuts. (NB: Recent research has shown an adverse effect on the colon mucosa of eating just 100g of peanuts a day for only five days. Production of the cells which line the colon wall increased by 20 per cent during that time. A rapid rate of cell division has been shown to be associated with increased risk of cancer).

FOODS TO FAVOUR
(FOODS IN BOLD ARE VERY BENEFICIAL)

Fruits; **vegetables**; pure fruit and vegetable juices, (and in particular seasonal fruits); apples and grapes; **onions**; **garlic**; Jerusalem artichokes; **sprouted seeds** and **beans**, such as mung beans; **beets**; **carrots**; peppers; **cucumbers**; **cabbage**; **watercress**; organic goats'/sheep's yoghurt; **whey and whey products**;

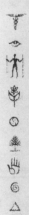

sauerkraut; **seaweeds**; foods made with miso; sourdough breads; apple cider vinegar; cereals and foods made from rye; **natural oats** and oat products; unpolished rice and rice products; barley and **millet**; almonds; hazelnuts; **pine nuts** and pumpkin seeds.

FAKE FOODS

A lot of things are taken by mouth that are not strictly foods, such as drugs, chewing gum (this interferes terribly with digestion), tea, coffee, laxatives and all calorie-free foods (such as soft drinks) which are therefore stimulating the digestive processes without any dietary benefits. Try to eliminate these false foods wherever possible from the diet, because eating them often leads to raised appetite levels which in turn leads to overeating. (Since the body does not get any food value out of them, they do not assuage hunger which is only really satisfied by nutritious foods.)

THE GOOD NEWS

NB: If 80 per cent of all food intake is sensibly chosen then the other 20 per cent is the margin – the enjoyment/festive/treat content which can normally be tolerated – which can also be health-sustaining because it lifts the spirits.

JUICING

Extracting juice from organic fruit and vegetables is one of the best ways to restore health and equilibrium to the colon. Investing in a good juicer will pay healthy dividends, and for purifying the system the following juices are known to be excellent: carrot, cabbage (a little only), celery, beetroot, apple and parsley.

As the food we eat is so tampered with today, and because of all the other pressures on body systems – environmental, stress-related, economic, dietary – it is wise to take this form of insurance protection, insurance that you are getting at least *some* of the vital nutrients you need daily. But the choice of vitamin supplements is bewildering. Also it is well known (to nutritional experts) that not all supplements are easily absorbed, either due to biological inadequacies caused by such factors as clogged colons and stressed digestive systems, or because the actual components of the supplements are not readily bio-available because the manufacturers have used forms which are cheaper in order to get a keener-priced product. The bottom line is you get what you pay for, so choose from a well-known supplier. However, there is a new range of vitamins on the market which are meant to be taken sub-lingually (under the tongue) and these may be useful for children and for those suffering from known dietary deficiencies as they by-pass the digestive tract altogether and are absorbed directly into the system. (See Useful Addresses for nutritional suppliers of all types of supplements.)

Try to take some form of fish oil supplement or evening primrose oil as well as vitamins and minerals. Follow the doses on the bottles unless advised otherwise. Keep all oil-based supplements in the refrigerator.

ADVICE FOR THE OVER-FORTIES AND THOSE WITH DIGESTIVE DIFFICULTIES

By the time one reaches the age of 40, gastric and other digestive juices are not so strong and enzyme production has also

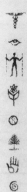

tailed off. Many people can help themselves by taking enzymes by mouth just before mealtimes, such as pineapple bromelain, papaya, betaine hydrochloride (for help in digesting proteins). Other, more specific enzymes can also be ordered for known deficiencies. Enzymes are not drugs but can produce near-magical effects if appropriately selected. Dosage is anything from 2–15 tablets taken 15–20 minutes before food but for anything more than 4 tablets per meal you should seek the sanction of a nutritional therapist, who can also advise about the more specific therapies available. Digestive enzymes may also control flatulence and wind.

EXAMINE THE OPTION OF FOOD COMBINING

There are many books on the market now which both explain the principles of food combining and offer recipes of how to go about it practically. (An excellent one appears in the Bibliography). Basically, this principle selects foods which are compatible with each other digestively, thus easing the strain on the digestive system. It also instructs in the balancing of acid and alkali-producing foods, a much-overlooked aspect of healthy nutrition. Many 'over forties' find food combining enables them to eat what they like through selecting correct combinations. Weight control is achieved by this process since the digestive system functions more effectively.

DEVELOPING A TRUE HUNGER INSTINCT

Re-training the digestive responses to indicate true hunger and not just boredom or the desire for a palliative 'warm drink' or chocolate may be difficult but will help with weight control. Examine your motives for wanting that which you are about to put into your mouth. Do you really need it? Or just want it? If you are having real problems with this aspect, keep beside you snacks that will sustain but not compromise your improved

condition, such as celery and carrot sticks, apple quarters,
cucumber slices, a few dried fruits, seeds or nuts, etc.

EATING WHEN STRESSED? TRY TO AVOID IT

Whoever invented business breakfasts should have their energies re-directed to re-constructing the health of those who have
suffered as a result. Digestion shuts down under stressful conditions so avoid anything which acts as an adverse stimulant
while eating. Television – especially the news – may be such a
factor. Try not to eat when upset. (NB: Unavoidable instances of
this are the perfect time to reach for the digestive enzymes to aid
nature.)

SUBSIDIARY CLEANSING TECHNIQUES

If you have undergone a course of colonic irrigation you have
begun, not ended, the process of cleansing your colon. It is
amazing how many people think they can undo the mistakes of
a lifetime in the twinkling of an eye. Consider a time factor of
3–6 months of concentrated effort and you may be getting
somewhere.

Meanwhile direct your efforts towards a variety of mini
programmes to further your cause, something that can be more
easily absorbed into daily life than an out-and-out nature cure.

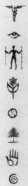

FOUR-DAY CLEANSE

This is basically designed to be used over a long weekend, one
of those boring winter ones where it is nice to know at the end
of it that something positive and useful has been achieved.

Strictly speaking, a three- or four-day programme is too short
to embark on a cleanse directed at the colon but is more effective if directed at resting and purifying the digestive system as
a whole.

Before you begin, have a day or two where you are watching

your diet, cutting down on heavier proteins and fats, tea, coffee and alcohol and concentrating on live fresh foods, grains and pulses.

Make sure that you are not constipated before beginning by taking a natural laxative, such as a teaspoon or two of linseed with plenty of water, or an extra helping (2–3 tablespoons) of oat bran. Prunes can also help your cause, as can an intestinal bulking agent, such as a teaspoon or two of psyllium husks in a large glass of water followed immediately by another glass (this is very important or you will become even more constipated). A mild herbal laxative may be preferred by some.

For your four-day cleanse eat only one kind of fruit. Choose from grapes, apples or plums (the latter only if you are habitually constipated). Buy the fruit in advance so that you are sure of a ripe supply of it and eat as much as you like. Drink plenty of water or mild herb teas but do not drink fruit juices. Abandon all vitamin therapy during the cleanse – you want your body to eliminate, not absorb.

Get to bed early and take a half-hour walk each day. Don't allow yourself to concentrate on problems. That's for later when you are fitter and better able to cope. Get back onto your regular diet slowly, taking a day or two to effect the transition, during which time you should eat only light foods, no animal produce and as many fresh foods as possible. Do this a few times each year and you will really begin to feel the difference.

MORE INTENSIVE BOWEL CLEANSES: THE SEVEN-DAY CLEANSE AND OTHERS

If you are envisaging a treatment as powerful as a seven-day cleanse you really should be doing so under the guidance of an expert in this field, since these often promote powerful healing reactions in which symptoms worsen for a time. Cleanses should not be attempted by anyone with an eating disorder or who is underweight, or who has been given a diet by their doctor. Anyone with a known health condition must get qualified professional advice before embarking on such a course.

Intensive bowel-cleansing courses utilize the same basic principles and they differ only slightly one from the other, though product names may confuse this similarity. They incorporate:

1   An intestinal bulking agent and lubricant such as psyllium husks, guar gum apple or citrus pectin. This acts like an intestinal broom.

2   An absorber of toxins which is usually volcanic ash or inert clay (usually bentonite) which acts like blotting paper.

3   A probiotic supplement containing acidophilus and sometimes other bowel flora to recolonize the bowel after the cleanse and replace any beneficial flora which may have been lost.

4   Herbal remedies, such as alfalfa or wheat grass, which cleanse by normalizing the electron balance in the colon.

5   Adjuncts to the above to help with the cleanse, such as a skin brush (for skin brushing *see Chapter 3*) or olive or castor oil for external application to abdomen.

This is a multi-faceted treatment, as are most holistic or complementary measures for restoring health. Quantities are increased as the cleanse progresses but these will vary from person to person, as will the rate at which the dose can be increased. Because only liquids are taken (besides the herbal preparations) they need to be done at a time when there are as few stresses as possible.

NB: Treatments like this are a very personal thing which is why no dosage recommendations or routines are included here:

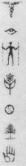

for these follow the guidelines of your cleansing programme or therapist. If following printed guidelines, be prepared to adapt these to your own conditional requirements.

The only other ingredient needed in addition to those mentioned above is willpower – yours – to stay on the liquid diet for a week. Some colonic irrigationists like to combine a seven-day cleanse with intensive colon hydrotherapy – a treatment a day. Others recommend the use of daily coffee enemas to stimulate the release of toxins from the liver as well as from the bowel.

NB: those who have never embarked on an intensive cleanse before should have a medical checkup first and follow an organized regime, ideally in a medically-supervised clinic licensed to operate such treatments.

That said, there are firm advocates for this type of regular (annual, bi-annual) intensive therapy, among them the now-famous Jason Winter, self-cured from terminal cancer (*see Bibliography*).

Green Farm offers an excellent do-it-yourself home colon cleansing pack to UK-based enquirers, consisting of fibre, herbs, skin-brushing equipment, stomach massage oil and pro-biotic supplements. Also available is an excellent booklet, *'Cleansing the Colon' (see Useful Addresses*). Any health hydro in the UK will implement similar routines when requested. In the USA there are specialist colon centres (*see Useful Addresses*), of which one of the best-known is Stanley Weinberger's Colon Health Centre. (Read *Healing Within* by the same expert). Other well-known bowel centres are those organized under the disciplines of Bernard Jensen and Norman Walker (enquire through their publishers).

THE SLOW CLEANSE

One of the most modern self-help methods of colon cleansing has been compiled by well-known US nutritional expert and herbalist Robert Gray, of Holistic Horizons. He has attempted to get around the very real problems presented to many people of taking time off from busy schedules in order to have an intensive cleanse, and his programme is designed to be incorporated into daily life without dieting, and it requires only a few minutes a day to implement – the time it takes to drink, twice daily, a glass of herbal preparation.

Basically the cleanse is done slowly over a period of up to three months, with the strength of the herbal products taken increasing as the cleanse proceeds. The person undergoing the cleanse stays in control of this process and progresses when they feel they are ready to go further. It is an excellent programme which I and several colleagues have tried personally. (See case histories in Chapter 7.) This is not to suggest it is favoured above other treatments mentioned above, simply well-suited to busy lifestyles (*see Useful Addresses*).

FUNCTIONAL BOWEL DISORDERS: TREATMENT SUGGESTIONS

The above therapeutic measures should go a long way towards setting in process the restoring of a normal bowel function, but in the meantime lingering or long-established bowel complaints may be helped by trying some of the measures noted here:

FLATULENCE (WIND) AND SIMPLE INDIGESTION

A simple glass of hot water can help. So can peppermint – add five drops of peppermint essence to hot water or drink it as tea. Or apply hot water externally (in a hot water bottle covered with a towel) to the stomach. With hyperacidity (acid rising in the mouth) Jan de Vries recommends the juice of a raw potato. First grate it, then squeeze out the juice and drink *immediately*.

Wind in the colon can sometimes be shifted by lying on the floor and raising the legs, hips and torso off the ground with the

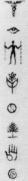

help of the arms (or a nearby wall) as support. Try a cycling movement with the legs in the air. Chewing a sprig of parsley also helps with wind.

Take nux vomica 6x if the indigestion is caused by over-indulgence.

Digestive enzymes often help.

SIMPLE CONSTIPATION (SEE ALSO CHAPTER 6)

Constipation is cured by following a simple formula – BLM – Bulk, Lubrication and Moisture. Put more fibre into the diet; use oat or rice bran in preference to wheat bran which can leach valuable minerals from the gut amongst other bad effects; drink more water. Hot water goes straight to the colon: drinking a glass of it first thing in the morning can be very stimulating for a sluggish bowel.

Use some oil, preferably olive oil on salads and for cooking. Take evening primrose or borage oil capsules, at least 500mg a day.

If you are on a slimming diet you must get BLM into your schedule despite this. Oat or rice bran is virtually calorie-free (drink with unsweetened grape juice, not milk). Or take psyllium husks, which are also calorie-free, with plenty of water! Lubrication can come from an olive oil and lemon dressing (very slimming) on the daily salad. Add garlic as this also tones the bowel.

Cabbage (add one tablespoon of finely chopped onion in the last five minutes of cooking for flavour) is a wonderful bulking agent for the bowel with cleansing and purifying properties as well. Avoid foods which bind the bowel, such as eggs, cheese, candies, white flour products, beef, coffee, salt and salted snack foods, fried foods, iron pills, chocolate, processed soups (even slimming soups) and stay off diuretics (unless prescribed by a doctor), antacids and antidepressants (ditto).

PRINCIPLES OF COLONIC IRRIGATION

NB: Laxatives and purgatives are *constipating* because in the end the bowel resists them and becomes even more stubborn.

PERSISTENT OR INTERMITTENT DIARRHOEA (IBS)

This type of diarrhoea often alternates with constipation and may have begun as a result of taking medication, such as antibiotics or pain-killers. It may be that the bowel is over-reacting to coming off medication before settling down. Take a well-balanced, wholefood, high fibre diet (experiment with fibres, if one type upsets you, try another). Rice bran oil usually helps considerably (*see Useful Addresses under Nutri-Centre*).

Stay off upsetting foods and have a blood test if food sensitivity is suspected. Try the following soothing remedy to control spasms: Mix 25g (1 oz) meadowsweet with 25g (1 oz) marshmallow root, 15g (½ oz) hops and 15g (½ oz) camomile flowers. Add this mixture to 1½l (3 pts) boiling water, cover and simmer for 15 minutes, allow to cool and strain. Take 3–4 tablespoons before each meal. If stress is a factor see Chapter 6.

DIVERTICULOSIS AND DIVERTICULITIS

The first is a functional disorder (*see Chapter 2*), the second a disease – a classic sign of the progression described in that chapter. Diverticula are little pockets (balloons in the bowel wall) which harbour faeces and thus can become infected (diverticulitis). As this is directly caused by constipation and the pressure which has been exerted to expel hard stools the remedy lies, as with constipation above, in BLM.

Analysis of stools belonging to sufferers indicates bread is the chief cause/culprit. And it is also advisable to stay off meat and dairy products and drink a glass of carrot juice a day (this helps the bowel lining to recover). Take plenty of Vitamin B complex and an acidophilus supplement between meals with water.

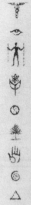

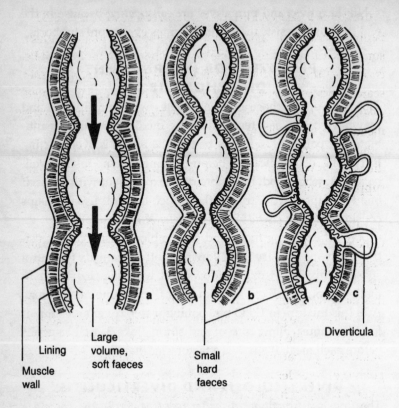

Muscle wall

Lining

Large volume, soft faeces

Small hard faeces

Diverticula

a   b   c

Colon muscles work best on a high-fibre diet but struggle to propel small volume faeces from a low fibre diet. Pressure on colon walls exerted by the strain may cause pouches (diverticula) to pop out. These then become stagnant breeding grounds for infection arising from decaying food.

Slippery elm gruel taken twice daily helps lubricate the stool, as does olive oil in the diet.

Homeopathic remedies may be helpful. Try nux vomica where there is an insufficient urge to go, silica where stools are difficult to expel and sulphur when the stools are large and painful to pass. Take all remedies to the 6x potency.

Serious, long-term inflammation-conditions of the intestines sometimes respond to eliminating certain foods thought to be corrosive from the diet. Naturopaths can help conduct this search with an exclusion diet or get a blood test (*see Useful Addresses*). Follow the dietary inclusions/exclusions recommended earlier in this chapter.

Acupuncture (*see Chapter 6*) can help balance the colon meridiens and is well-worth trying. Conventional treatment tends to suppress symptoms, not get to causes.

CANCER OF THE COLON AND/OR RECTUM

Cancer is a disease of the immune system which has, at some stage in the past, failed to recognize rogue cancer cells which crop up from time to time in routine cell division. No conventional treatment will apply itself to this factor and the only way to do so is to build up the general health and resistance. Take 6–12 glasses of pure vegetable juice daily, especially carrot, and drink within minutes of preparation; become vegetarian, (under professional guidance) consider carefully before allowing yet more toxins to enter your body in the form of chemotherapy, read books such as Dr Max Gerson's *Cancer Therapy: Results of Fifty Cases*, and THINK. Investigate other pioneers and their natural cures.

Don't try to rush any elimination process: toxins caused by and causing the disease must be eliminated in the controlled way. Don't accept your fate or what you're told to do – find out all your options.

NB: Stomach and duodenal ulcers, hiatus hernia, ileitis, and malabsorption conditions such as pernicious anaemia and coeliac disease, all of which can and do affect digestive function, are not really within the scope of this book. However, the publishers of this book produce excellent titles devoted to those conditions – some of which are listed in the Bibliography.

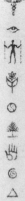

CANDIDA AND INTESTINAL PARASITES: CAUSES AND CURES

Candida used to be more commonly known as a woman's Christian name: now it is a complaint on everyone's lips.

Yet despite its widespread recognition as such, very little is understood about it. In fact, it is the organism underlying increasingly prevalent complaints such as thrush, which may appear in the mouth, vagina, under the nails, between the toes and in sweaty parts of the skin. But its chief site is in the colon – any other appearance is caused by an invasion from the colon due to imbalanced conditions in secondary organs.

Candida belongs to the fungal family, which are plants that can't make their own food because they have no chlorophyll or green colouring. It is therefore a parasite, an opportunistic organism that feeds upon its host. In fact it is one of the observed 400 different species of organisms which have been identified in the human gut.

What makes it so dangerous to colon health is that it is a dimorphic organism. In its single-cell form it is known as a type of yeast, but it also has a fungal form which produces branches and can put down roots. These roots, like any plant root system, can become very invasive and penetrate seemingly impenetrable barriers. Unfortunately candida is capable of penetrating the colon walls which is potentially lethal to good health,

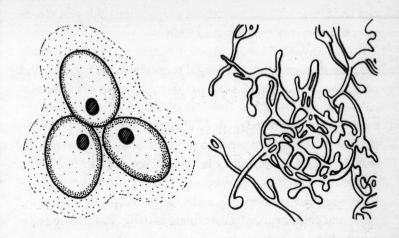

Simple candida cells.

Invasive candida cell showing tendrils. These can penetrate bowel walls.

because in ideal health colon walls act as a barrier, keeping the putrefying and, sometimes undesirable, contents of the gut out of general blood circulation to the rest of the body. Such a semi-permeable barrier should allow only nutrients through its walls to sustain the life of its host, not undesirables.

In normal health, candida is kept under control by other competing organisms, so that it is never able to get out of hand. But modern junk-food diets and unhealthy, sedentary lifestyles are favouring the conditions it prefers and threatening those held by protective organisms such as lactobacillus. Other contemporary factors which favour its overgrowth are antibiotics (which wipe out good, controlling bacteria like acidophilus as well as the 'bad' ones they were prescribed to treat, but don't touch fungi at all), the pill (which creates a hormonal climate candida loves), cortico-steroids such as those

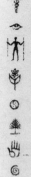

PRINCIPLES OF COLONIC IRRIGATION

given for arthritis (and some skin disorders) and certain chemicals used in foods and household preparations. Air and chemical pollution may contribute as well.

All or any of these produce a climate in which candida assumes its more virulent, fungal form which, as it grows and penetrates the intestinal walls, causes toxins from its own metabolic processes AND the contents of the gut to escape into the main system and bloodstream. When this happens not only are its spores conveyed to other parts of the body (vagina, mouth, skin, etc) to set up secondary infections, but also escaped toxins compromise body cell metabolism, causing a variety of symptoms which are so confusing and so apparently unrelated to the colon and colon health that treatment usually totally ignores the cause of the problem – and therefore is both inadequate and ineffectual in the long term. No cure can ever be achieved unless the true cause of the complaint is known and treated.

Thus sufferers of thrush can take long courses of antifungals such as nystan or even the stronger varieties such as ketoconazole or fluconazole (sold under a variety of brand names) and even though there is an improvement while they are being taken the condition never quite clears up, and usually becomes progressively more and more difficult to treat.

Furthermore, immune system reactions occur, because part of the contents which seep through the colon walls will be partially-digested proteins which the immune system recognizes as foreign invaders. Thus, over a long-term period, the immune system can become exhausted, firstly by having to fight the fungus and keep its numbers down, secondly by reacting against the toxins and, thirdly, against the foreign invaders.

No wonder one of the chief of many symptoms associated with this complaint is tiredness, lethargy and susceptibility to minor infections. No wonder it has been said that systemic, untreated candidiasis (the official name of the complaint arising from a candida infection) carries a 100 per cent mortality rate. No wonder that nearly every serious illness in its terminal stages is made more complex with candidiasis, from cancer to Aids. But the sobering thought is not that such diseases *end up* with candida, but that they may, at least in part, be *caused* by it and the havoc it wreaks with the immune system. Most ME sufferers have candidiasis.

DIAGNOSING AND ACKNOWLEDGING THE THREAT

It is said that candida is so difficult to diagnose positively that often the diagnosis only occurs as a result of successful treatment; in other words if the sufferer gets better as a result of the treatment, then it is likely that candida was the underlying cause. So if candidiasis is suspected, it is wise to try the treatment rather than wait to establish positive diagnosis, since the treatment will not do any harm whether candida is the problem or not.

Looking at the following symptoms, all of which are associated with candida overgrowth, will illustrate the difficulty: (NB: as listed by Stanley Weinberger from the Colon Health Centre near San Francisco, in his excellent book about colon health called *Healing Within*. These are things he has seen in his work in the clinic which is one of the few to recognize the real threat to health from candida and other parasites – see page 94).

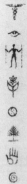

Central Nervous system disorders: depression, anxiety, irrational irritability, lethargy, fatigue, agitation, inability to concentrate, memory loss and headaches, including migraines.

Intestinal disorders: bloating, diarrhoea, constipation, heartburn, gastritis, indigestion and colitis.

Allergic manifestations: severe chemical and food sensitivities, asthma, acne, hives, sinusitis, hay fever, skin rashes, earaches and possibly psoriasis.

Add to this list those lifted from a selection of self-diagnosis leaflets for those suspecting they have candidiasis (mentioned elsewhere by Weinberger):

Anal and vulval itching, vaginal discharge (usually white) burning and tearing of eyes, nasal twitching, runny nose, muscle weakness, numbness, skin burning or tingling, feeling spacey or unreal, muscle aches, joint pains, tightness in the lungs (sometimes with white expectorant), rashes, wind, dry mouth, burning on urination, urinary frequency, failing vision, recurrent infections or fluid in ears, prostratitis, impotence, loss of sexual desire.

Is it any wonder doctors call it the humbug diagnosis?

Evidence that candidiasis is increasingly prevalent persists, despite medical scepticism. On good days sufferers feel fine; they feel just like they should always be feeling. What seems to happen on those good days is that for one reason or another, the immune system is coping better than usual with controlling the fungus. Just how vital the immune system is to health has been explained elsewhere.

Obviously something must be done to control candida's overgrowth, before a vicious circle is created whereby vitamin and mineral deficiencies (created by the excessive demand of the candida organism to sustain its own growth) lead on to enzyme deficiencies (enzymes are manufactured from vitamins). This will, in turn, further weaken the immune system, since it relies on enzymes for its first line of defence.

Apart from physicians' prescriptions for antifungals, such as Nystatin, well worth trying so long as other measures to improve resistance are implemented, other treatments have to be self-administered on a see-if-I-feel-better basis. If a prescription has been refused because your symptoms are too vague, you may like to try the safe antifungal caprylic acid, which is derived from coconut, and take it for at least a month according to directions on the bottle. NB: If vaginal thrush co-exists, try also tea-tree pessaries, which may have to be inserted at night (vaginally) for the same length of time.

The next measures are all dietary. Firstly, cut out all foods that may contain live moulds and yeasts, such as beer, wine, cider, ketchup, mustard, cheese, sour cream, buttermilk, commercial yoghurts,[1] mushrooms, vinegar, pickles, sour milk, soy sauce, miso, tofu, vegetable extracts. Next, sweets and sugar have to go as the yeast thrives on it. This means sugar, honey, molasses, maple syrup (even artificial sweeteners are thought to aggravate candida so this is an excellent time to break yourself from these chemicals, for that is what they are, not foods). Fruits and juices will have to go too, however pure, and because of the moulds on them, dried fruit.

Another group of foods to which candida sufferers are particularly sensitive are processed meats. This means any meats that are cured, dried or smoked, also fish treated in a similar way. Luncheon meats, sausages and frankfurters, corned beef, pastrami, burgers and all pork products, should be abandoned for a period of one month (preferably forever).

Beverages: Besides those mentioned above do not drink any gassy drinks at all, including low calorie varieties. All caffein-

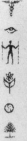

---

[1] Commercial yoghurts rarely contain live acidophilus to the strength that would be considered effective by bowel therapists.

PRINCIPLES OF COLONIC IRRIGATION

containing drinks (tea, coffee, cocoa) will have to be sacrificed. Saké and spirits had best be excluded as alcohol is very closely allied to sugar and its effects.

If this seems totally unacceptable, depressing and impossible to follow, consider the very substantial list of foods you can eat: lamb, poultry, a little beef (try to get organic meat so it doesn't contain chemicals, antibiotics or hormones), fish, eggs, fresh vegetables, unsalted butter, low-fat natural live goats' or sheep's yoghurt and low-fat milk.

Of seeds, nuts, legumes and grains you can eat brown rice and whole grains, as well as almonds, sunflower seeds and pumpkin seeds (good on cereals of which you can choose between corn, buckwheat, millet and rice for preference as they are lower in gluten (candida-sensitive) than other cereals, but make sure they are not sweetened and keep the carbohydrate content of food down. (Just for this period it is almost essential to favour a high protein diet – but eat plenty of salads and green vegetables with the protein.)

Olive oil, spices, and herbs are unlimited, as are garlic and onions. Garlic is a great antifungal and can be taken in capsule form if not liked in food. Lemons are the only fruits which are acceptable at this time.

Canned foods are not favoured but certain emergency supplies can be eaten from time to time, such as tuna, sardines and water chestnuts (which make an interesting texture/taste variation). A few canned tomatoes and tomato paste is acceptable. Basically the rule is: avoid additives, fungi, fermented products (such as vinegar and beer), sugar or sugar substitutes.

Wholemeal flour and products made from it, such as bread, as well as pasta and pastry, seem to be acceptable to some sufferers, as the yeast used to raise the flour is cooked and therefore dead, but basically it is wise to stick to crispbreads since so many candida sufferers are wheat and yeast sensitive whether the products are cooked or not.

Herb teas may be drunk as may dandelion coffee. One of the best teas to drink is pau d'arco (lapacho), because of its antifungal properties. Lapacho capsules can also be taken and may prove very helpful as lapacho is a powerful antifungicide. (*See Rio Trading in Useful Addresses.*)

COLON CLEANSING

During the four weeks that you are trying this exclusion diet, it is an option worth considering to try a course of colonic irrigation, whereby the therapist can give implants which will help balance the intestinal flora. The cleansing action may initially stir up the candida but with concentrated attention to diet, etc, plus the regular taking of antifungals by mouth, the effect can enhance your efforts. One treatment, at the most two a week, is the norm, anything more intensive must be ordered by a health expert specializing in the treatment of candida.

THE DIE-OFF REACTION

This phenomenon, known as the Herxheimer reaction, can lead to temporarily unpleasant symptoms which have all the characteristics of a reaction to a toxic substance. This is in fact a good sign since it means large numbers of yeast cells are dying, but unfortunately in so doing they are releasing their toxins into the bloodstream. Symptoms include many of those you have come to associate with bad days with the candida infection, such as itching, headaches, nausea, muscular aches and flu-like symptoms.

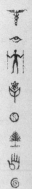

Rest and drink plenty of water to help flush out the toxins and if they become particularly severe, stop the antifungal medications for a day or two until they have settled down. Reactions such as this make it essential for you to have made contact with your physician or qualified health expert so that your progress can be monitored. You may have had to suffer candida alone but do not suffer the treatment without qualified supervision.

If the treatment has helped you but symptoms return after the month is up, you need longer. Watch carefully for adverse reactions when you re-introduce certain foods into your diet – it may be that you will have to exclude certain of them for the forseeable future.

PRESERVING COLON HEALTH WITH PROBIOTICS

Anyone who has had, and learned to control, candida learns to live a much healthier life, and usually continues to avoid foods which have been artificially packaged, processed, canned, coloured and flavoured, since they all contain additives on which candida thrives. Even the packaging itself intrudes into the food and superimposes its range of chemicals on the contents. Besides these caveats, consider very carefully before taking any medication or antibiotic treatment, since not only are those fake foods – even something as 'harmless' as aspirin has no sustaining/supportive value to the body, it is an intruder – but also they are likely to do as much harm as good.

The new antibiotics are probiotics, meaning they are FOR life, not against it. In this remarkable new armoury against disease come items which the average person would never consider to be disease-resisting entities, such as food itself, especially partitioned foods, ie foods from which certain elements have been extracted or concentrated in order to achieve a more powerful effect.

Numbered among such foods are *amino acids*, the building blocks of the body. Derived from natural foodstuffs, in this case proteins, selected aminos can help put you to sleep at night, wake you up, protect you from exhaustion, build you up for peak physical performance – whatever . . . yet they are FOODS, not fake foods. Amino acid therapy is one of the tools of future health.

Vitamins and *minerals* also come into this category and large therapeutic doses of vitamins have been seen to be more effective against some established diseases than antibiotics, chemotherapy or any of the medications the drug companies care to concoct.

Enzymes are also increasingly being used to aid digestion, facilitate absorption of food where difficulties are encountered and generally help those who are having difficulties in some or other of life's processes. This therapy is of especial value to the over-forties, since enzyme production slows down after that and may cause problems with digestion, elimination, absorption etc. All these are foods, *not drugs*, being used in specific ways and in strengths needed to bring about an effect.

INTESTINAL FLORA:
FEEDING YOUR INTERNAL GARDEN

One of the most exciting and effective ways to protect and sustain colon health is by taking intestinal flora supplements, since these are now seen to have an 'antibiotic' effect on alien organisms in the gut. Introducing large quantities of these helpful organisms sustains the body's natural defences but does not interfere with the way in which natural reactions to foreign invaders takes place. Hence their action is *pro*biotic – for health, but their effect is *anti*biotic – against microbes.

Care must be taken when selecting live supplements for the colon and digestive system, as many opportunists, seeing a growth market, are introducing products which may seem to be bona fide but in fact have about as much biological/food value as a baby's dummy. Thus there are many lactobacillus acidophilus supplements on the market which are not derived from human strains and therefore not thought to be as effective.

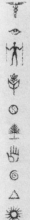

In a survey conducted several years ago in Britain, the leading UK health magazine, the *Journal of Alternative and Complementary Medicine*, reported that from some 30 acidophilus products tested, only three had any viable flora. Suspect any products which do not come from well-known reliable sources, which haven't got a very short shelf life, which don't need refrigeration after opening (not *all* good supplements require this but most recommend it. Use them quickly.) Another way of tackling the potency problem with acidophilus supplements is to raise your own. US expert Robert Gray gives a recipe in his excellent book, *The Colon Health Handbook* which is reproduced here with his permission.

Robert Gray points out that the lactobacteria we eat are present in milk and come from the vegetable matter eaten by cows. Cabbage is one vegetable that is teeming with lactobacteria – that is one reason why it is so good for us when raw. We can make lactobacteria without a starter from cabbage as follows:

Blend together 1¾ cups (420 ml) distilled or purified water plus 3 cups (720 ml) coarsely chopped, loosely packed, fresh cabbage, plus ⅛th teaspoon (½ml) of dry, granulated garlic. Start the blender at low speed, and then advance to high speed and blend for more than 30 seconds. Pour into a jar, cover and let stand at room temperature for three days. At this time, strain off the liquid rejuvelac. This initial batch of cabbage rejuvelac takes three days to make, but succeeding batches take only 24 hours. Each morning, after straining off the fresh rejuvelac, blend together 1½ cups (360 ml) distilled or purified water plus 3 cups (720 ml) of coarsely chopped, loosely-packed fresh cabbage, plus ⅛th teaspoon (½ ml) of dry, granulated garlic for 30 seconds at high speed. Pour into a jar, add ¼ cup (60 ml) of the fresh rejuvelac which has just been strained off, cover, shake and let stand at room temperature until next morning.

You can also make cabbage rejuvelac without a blender by

chopping the cabbage very finely and using 2½ cups (600 ml) finely-chopped, closely packed fresh cabbage for every 3 cups (720 ml) finely-chopped, freshly packed, cabbage listed above. The amount of distilled or purified water should remain unchanged. Good quality rejuvelac tastes similar to a cross between carbonated water and the whey obtained when making yoghurt. Never consume the rejuvelac if it has a putrid odour. NB: Gray says that some environments require a negative ion generator in the room where the rejuvelac is being made to inhibit harmful bacteria.

Drink each day's quantity of rejuvelac during the course of the day, dividing it into three doses, taken preferably with meals. Always discard any not consumed within 24 hours. Refrigerate once prepared.

Although there are supplements on the market which contain diverse strains of lactobaccillus and sometimes streptococcus as well, which may be bona fide, it is thought to be preferable to take each strain separately, taking one type for one month, then changing to the other.

When (ie what time of day) these supplements are taken is also important for their successful implantation in the colon. Take lactobacillus acidophilus away from food, with water only, as otherwise the flora will never survive the journey through the stomach and small intestine.

There is a strain of acidophilus available in America which is acid-resistant. Called DDS-1 Acidophilus, it is available from the Colon Health Centre, near San Francisco, California (*see Useful Addresses*). Solgar also do excellent nutritional aids of all kinds (available in the UK and in the USA where they are manufactured). In the top three in Britain for acidophilus potency came a product by Biocare; they also specialize in enzymes and their address is in the Useful Addresses section.

In an excellent little booklet, *The Friendly Bacteria*, author

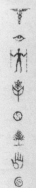

William H. Lee (*see Bibliography*) points out that lactobacillus bulgaricus should be taken with meals as its action is through the lymph network and therefore it has to go through the digestive process. (This does not have to be of human strain to be effective.) All these substances will become the new 'medicine' of the twenty-first century. They all follow the basic health premise so forgotten by contemporary medicine and its drugs: *first do no harm*.

NATURAL WAYS OF INCREASING INTESTINAL FORTITUDE

Ancient cultures have usually developed health-protecting measures and so it is not surprising to find that products rich in lactobacillus activity have traditionally been made and used in countries known for longevity such as Bulgaria. These include yoghurt made from lactobacillus bulgaricus; from India, kefir – a yoghurt-like food fermented with lactobacillus: from Japan, miso; from Western Europe, cheese; and from Germany, sauerkraut. Such foods produce lactic acid which is known to be beneficial to colon health as this provides the right environment for protective flora to implant and prosper. It also helps provide the right pH in the bowel, which in itself is a protection since Candida will not flourish in such an environment.

Thus home-made yoghurt, made with *fresh* milk, is an excellent way to protect against the unseen invaders of the gut. NB: All fermented products should be consumed within 24 hours of opening/making otherwise their efficacy wanes and by-products which the bacteria produce may become too profuse.

KOMBUCHA: NECTAR OF THE GODS

Another fermented drink which is prized for health due to both its oxygen-producing qualities and its ability to metabolize acids valued to the colon and digestive system, since they help to deal with toxins, is Kombucha, a drink made from tea which has been used in Japan for centuries and is also widely drunk now in Germany.

The same as with the kefir fungus, it is made with a sprouting fungus possessing antibiotic properties. In the course of working on the tea (and sugar dissolved therein) the fungus produces glucuronic acid, which is thought to form compounds with metabolic waste products as well as substances alien to the body (drugs and toxins) which aid in detoxification. Lactic acid is also produced and helps balance intestinal flora, but the main advantage is thought to come from its production of the glucoronic acid which is a component of vital body tissues, in particular the gastric mucous membranes.

Since 1964 Kombucha has enjoyed a tremendous revival due to the research of Dr Rudolf Skelnar, a German physician who researched its effects on cancer patients for more than thirty years and found that the fungus' effects on cancer cells was powerfully remedial.

Already-brewed Kombucha can be purchased in some health food stores, but it is so easy to 'brew' that the best way is to make enquiries about how to get a starter fungus: then the remedy can be produced for a few pence a day – in sufficient quantities for a household. It is naturally carbonated through the fermentation process and extremely pleasant to drink. A book has been published about the research which has been conducted, mainly in Germany (*see Bibliography*): the instructions of how to brew it are always passed on with the fungus. Many alternative cancer centres and colonic irrigationists have heard of it and may know where to obtain it. There is an address in Useful Addresses from which access to information and Kombucha products may be obtained.

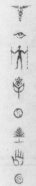

Stanley Weinberger, in his book *Healing Within*, draws our attention to a further largely unrecognized enemy to health – parasites. He quotes statistics that show that in certain areas of the world more than 80 per cent of the population has parasites, and it is not just a problem of third world countries either: in North America alone, he says, at least 21 million people are afflicted.

This major threat to health was recognized in the 1912 meeting in London of 57 leading UK physicians mentioned earlier in chapter 3. But since then, like a sleeping giant, recognition of the threat to health has remained dormant – until the last decade or two, when the frequency and availability of travel to remote areas of the world has caused a tremendous influx of people to be infected with all kinds of parasites, from guardia (a waterborne parasite which is believed to have now reached epidemic proportions) to the more common types of worms, including tapeworms, pinworms, hookworms, ringworms, roundworms – some of them a few inches long, others as much as 30 feet long. Of course, they live in the colon and the unhealthier this is the easier they find it to survive and breed, dumping their toxic wastes, like candida, into the bloodstream of their host.

The most common of these are pinworms and it is estimated that one in five children in the general population of temperate climates have them. They infect the lower bowel and rectum and often cause anal itching at night. They feed primarily on sweets and refined carbohydrates, which induces a further craving for these foods.

Tapeworms are also common and can be got from poorly cooked meats and fish and from animal faeces. Worms can be passed from handling pets and children must be taught to wash their hands after patting or playing with animals.

The tremendous increase in the incidence of tapeworms in America is thought to be caused by the increase in demand for rare and raw beef. But it is contaminated pork that presents the largest threat to health, because the animals are so commonly infected with parasites (such as balatidium) which can be passed directly to the gut of humans.

Unfortunately, the symptoms of having parasites can be confused with many other illnesses and infections so many people remain undiagnosed. Colonic irrigation can be a great advantage here if parasites are suspected, since 25 varieties of them can be seen with the naked eye and detection through the viewing tube during the colonic is often the way by which positive diagnosis is made.

THE CAECUM: FERMENTATION POUCH

Between the small and large intestines is a valve, the ileo-caecal valve, through which largely digested food passes into the first part of the colon or large intestine, the caecum. The bag-like structure caecum has been likened to the leather pouches traditionally used by wandering tribes for bacterial fermentation of fresh milk products into yoghurts – the design being perfect for the encouragement of such activities.

Unfortunately, the caecum's design, perfect for the natural fermentation of digested food in the final stages of its transformation into faeces, is also a perfect harbour for parasites. The importance of keeping bowel contents moving is given further emphasis by this factor; also it is important to ensure that the valve between the small and large intestines is in good working order. If pain, discomfort or bloating is experienced in the lower, right-hand quadrant of the abdomen, suspect caecal problems and massage (for twenty seconds only) one or other of the acupressure points shown on the diagram. Avoid gum-chewing and teeth-grinding, as these two habits can affect the

110

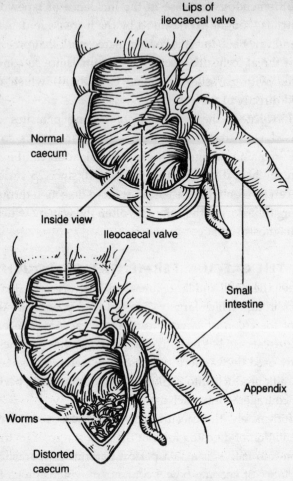

Lips of
ileocaecal valve

Normal
caecum

Inside view

Ileocaecal valve

Small
intestine

Appendix

Worms

Distorted
caecum

Contents from small intestine (above) flow into the caecum via the ileocaecal valve.

functioning of this valve and so affect the activities in the caecum. The appendix protects the caecum from infection and should never be removed unless absolutely necessary.

If you have been abroad, especially to countries like Africa or India and have returned with intestinal symptoms you did not

PRINCIPLES OF COLONIC IRRIGATION

have before, suspect parasites. Ask your doctor to test for guardia, gardnarella and other bowel infections.

Never take the possibility of parasite infections lightly: one booklet about them describes their effects thus: 'Parasites are vermin that steal your food, drink your blood and leave their excrement in your body to be reabsorbed into the bloodstream as nourishment.'

THE HUMBLE WALNUT AND OTHER ANTI-PARASITIC REMEDIES

A tincture made from walnuts is one of the most powerful of remedies against intestinal parasites. In America Stanley Weinberger of the previously-mentioned Colon Health Centre uses a product known as K-Min, and also recommends castor oil capsules, but taken in a special way – frozen – otherwise, he says, they will not reach the part of the intestine where the worms are, but would be absorbed into the system too early.

The ingredients mentioned in regard to colon cleansing are also excellent since they sweep the intestines and scour and cleanse the encrusted colon walls which harbour the parasites. Another remedy often prescribed by herbalists is wormwood.

Together with these a general cleanser such as wheat grass is recommended. Alfalfa, wheat grass, chlorella and spirulina are all excellent 'green' products which help clean the intestines. The chlorophyll they contain has an antiseptic effect on colon walls, besides providing valuable minerals and nutrients. Fresh garlic is another wonderful antiseptic.

As well as these measures the implants given during colonic irrigations can be invaluable for introducing cleansing and toning substances to the bowel. A great favourite of well-known bowel expert, David Webster, is to use irrigation to introduce a high-grade, strong acidophilus strain (as many as 50 billion) into the colon plus implants of whey, which acidifies the bowel,

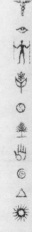

PRINCIPLES OF COLONIC IRRIGATION

helps the acidophilus 'to take', by providing it with the right environment, and kills parasites because they do not like the acid environment provided by these two ingredients. Webster says that two or three treatments of this nature will diminish the total number of colonics needed (the whey must be freshly-prepared) whilst repopulating the bowel with healthy flora. (See *Acidophilus and Colon Health* by David Webster.)

Care of the colon by as many means as are necessary, can protect you from a variety of potentially lethal and partially unsuspected complaints and conditions which could, if not confronted, lead on to progressive states of disease.

COLON CONSCIOUSNESS:
THE MANAGEMENT
OF STRESS

Psychologists tell us that that which is buried and unacknowledged in our lives is that which is likely to cause complexes, leading to all kinds of physical and psychological symptoms which emerge during the stressful times of life to haunt us until we find out their cause and do something about them.

The increase in the incidence of IBS and other digestive complaints, not all of which have identifiable physical causes, leads us to the inevitable conclusion that the widespread dysfunction of the bowel which we as a society are experiencing, may in part have its roots in unconscious stresses and problems associated with our contemporary mores and lifestyles.

C. Leslie Thomson, a Scot who was ahead of his time and the author of *Constipation and our Civilisation* earlier this century wrote: 'In life there are two ways of avoiding discomfort: the modern way is to produce sensory paralysis. The natural way is to live so that pain is unnecessary.' He also said, 'cures are not for sale.'

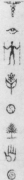

THE COLON AND
ITS REACTION TO STRESS

Turning once more to colloquial language we find many reinforcements to the acknowledged link between the digestive system and the bowel and the central nervous system and the brain, especially those parts of it which are beyond conscious control. Thus we have phrases such as 'sick to the stomach', 'something is eating me', 'this turns my stomach, gnaws at my vitals, gives me the shits'. We have descriptive phrases linking the emotion of fear with the digestive processes – 'gnawing fear, butterflies in the stomach'; and anger – 'my gorge rises'. All these phrases suggest that digestive processes are compromised in some way by such emotions, and in reverse we find that strength of digestion is described by phrases which express courage and rightness, 'he's got guts'; 'my gut reaction tells me . . . .'

Science reinforces the link expressed by language. Speaking of the bowel and stress John Northover, Consultant Surgeon at St Marks Hospital (London) for Diseases of the Rectum and Colon said:

'the bowel is a very complex piece of our anatomy and the nerve supply to it is very complex indeed with connections to pretty well every other part of you. The bowel is receiving messages from the brain and spinal cord all the time – vast numbers of messages, and if you're stressed or something else is happening then that will have an effect on the rate at which the bowel muscle is contracting, the rate at which things move on.'

THE HARA: VITAL CENTRE OF MAN

Ancient cultures confirm their belief in this link between psyche and soma (or physical body) and attempt to explain it through

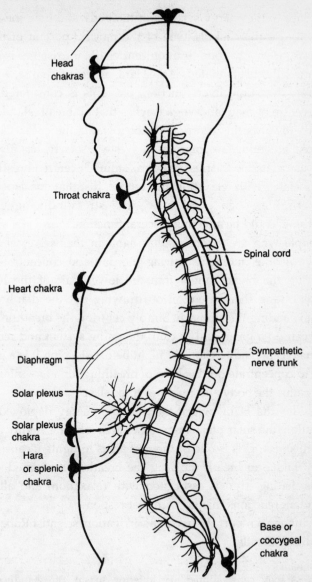

Sites of the seven main chakras (or energy configuration points) on the body, of which the vitality of the second (hara) or splenic chakra is vital to digestive health and function.

reference to the energy systems of the body and how they are organized – the chakras. One of the most important of these chakras, or energy-configuration centres (their existence is now scientifically substantiated) is the Hara, or second chakra, which controls digestion, liver function, etc. This is considered the vital centre of man, and yoga teaches that all breath should be drawn towards this centre and not towards the chest. Chest-centred breathing, so common in Western society, has always been associated with stress, whereas stomach-centred breathing is associated with relaxation and repose. Just that one aspect of Western life, yoga experts say, the stress-inducing chest breathing, could be affecting visceral function.

People who are aware of that habit in themselves should pause in quiet moments during the day and concentrate on drawing the breath down into the lower part of the body, concentrating their attention on drawing out the diaphragm and expanding the stomach. Simply centring the breath in this way can do a great deal to calm the entire system and reduce apprehension and tension. At night before sleeping it is a good idea to concentrate on this kind of breathing for a few minutes, as it calms the body and prepares it for sleep.

Besides the Hara, which controls the energy deployed for digestion, the solar plexus is another area which is highly reactive to stress. This is one of the first areas to tighten, causing a sharp intake of breath (holding the breath is associated with stress, letting it go is associated with relaxation) and all the attendant reactions that go with that response.

Writing in a report about colonic irrigation, scientist Robert C. Kelvinson details:

'stress may cause alimentary anterior spasm. Stress-induced hypoxia often manifests in the descending colon due to inadequacies in anastomosis that supply the splenic flexure . . . When a critical level of tissue damage is reached (dependent on faecal chemistry, temperature etc) further destruction precipitates by bacteria within the lumen.'

In lay language what this means is that stress upsets bowel function which in turn (and in time) allows the destructive bacteria in the gut to gain hold and begin breaking down the bowel walls. Alterations in physical structure such as this can only lead on to disease.

In *Healing Within*, Stanley Weinberger describes this process graphically:

'Over a period of time, if the colon loses its ability to have a regular, rhythmic peristaltic flow its nerve signals stop functioning and large deposits of waste gradually lodge in its many pockets and convolutions. This waste paralyses the ileo-caecal valve, backs up into the small intestine, and is re-absorbed into the bloodstream. Parasites as well as bacteria flourish in this environment. Once the colon's flexures (turns) are plugged, it cannot support peristaltic action, it loses its "memory" and no longer functions in a normal way.'

He goes on to say that the three major causes of such dysfunction are emotional stress, improper dietary habits and subconscious complexes to do with such things as toilet training or negative attitudes or anxiety about one's body functions.

It is one thing to know about something and another to learn how to deal with it. First the cause of stress has to be isolated, then treated with whatever therapeutic approach seems appropriate. This chapter contains a variety of suggestions for dealing with stress, but in the first place it may be helpful to examine stress's more common manifestations on the bowel, which may have ramifications on weight, or be nerve-related, or cause

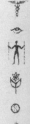

functional disorders, such as decreasing or increasing peristalsis, or lead to imbalances in one of the three stages of processing food, ie digestion, absorption and elimination. NB: It is more common today to find imbalances due to faulty elimination than to the two previous stages of digestion, simply because we in the West eat too much, too often and give too little heed to food content, so that body energies are constantly directed towards digestion and assimilation and away from the vital process of elimination.

STRESS AND WEIGHT CONTROL

Being both underweight and overweight are disease-states, just as alcoholism is a disease state. There is, within certain parameters, a normal weight for each and every one of us, tied to age, height and bone structure. To deviate more than a few kilograms from this weight is a sign that the body is imbalanced, due either to mental imbalances affecting food intake, or physical (metabolic) imbalances probably due to diet. 'Where the mind goes, the body follows', and some interesting observations have been made in connection with both physiognomy (face structure) and posture. These apparently give the game away to certain experts who have been studying people trying to lose (or in rare cases gain) weight for many decades. (It is a sign of our times that rarely are we trying to gain weight).

DIAGNOSIS BY POSTURE

To gain an early insight into what a lifetime of eating habits may have done to your anatomical shape, consider your self sideways in the mirror before dressing one morning. Stand in a relaxed way. Any deviation from normal posture (sway-back, tummy protruberances, 'duck' posture etc) points to damaged digestive organs, says Erich Rauch, MD, proponent of the

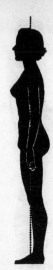

1. Normal posture. Line shows relationship to centre of gravity.

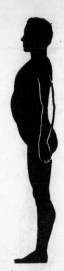

2. Abnormal posture: 'Attention'. The overstuffed stomach/ intestines need more room and so forward distortion occurs.

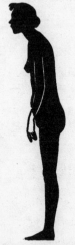

3. Abnormal posture: 'Head start'. Intestinal slackness causes downward and forward abdominal and spinal displacement.

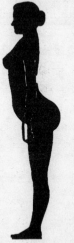

4. Abnormal posture: 'The duck'. The enlarged abdomen leads to a backward displacement of the pelvis and buttocks.

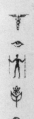

PRINCIPLES OF COLONIC IRRIGATION

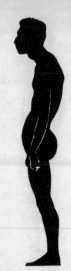

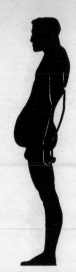

5. Abnormal posture: 'Lazybones'. Glutted intestines, together with poor musculature, cause slumping.

6. Abnormal posture: 'The sower'. Severe intestinal slackness plus unexpelled faeces prompt lower belly bagging.

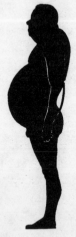

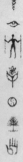

7. Abnormal posture: 'The bass drum player'. The tremendous increase in abdominal contents may be due to gas and faeces retention.

Illustrations reproduced from 'Health through inner body cleansing' by Erich Rauch, M.D. with kind permission from Editions Haug International.

PRINCIPLES OF COLONIC IRRIGATION

famous Mayr School of Intestinal Therapy in Europe. Rauch believes that because of the sheer volume of the intestines (30 feet in all) they will, over the years, if glutted or allowed to get slack, take over more and more space in the abdomen, pushing other organs out of the way and ultimately causing the spine to grow into a position to accommodate this invasion.

The way in which this happens is a sign of what specifically has caused it, for example the typical retired army officer figure usually stands to attention with the chest out and the tummy held high 'to attention'. Rauch says this is a sign of a habitually over-stuffed stomach. Those who tend to lean forward as they walk, or slump into themselves tend to suffer from slack intestines with little muscular force etc. Those with a 'duck' posture (bottom waggling at the back when they walk) have a greatly enlarged abdomen which has over the years re-positioned the pelvis.

Most people have a fair idea what it is they do, or neglect to do, and self-examination of this kind often brings the result of many years of such habits to the forefront of consciousness where they can be (1) acknowledged and (2) tackled.

THE TYRANNY OF SLENDERNESS

There is a definite connection between slimming and bowel disorders, which is why women suffer far more frequently from IBS and constipation than men. In fact recent statistics show that over 90 per cent of women have at some stage in their lives been on a diet. In 1–2 per cent this develops into full-blown anorexia by the time they are 16–18; in 20 per cent it develops into a pattern of 'binge' eating usually once a month of which 2–3 per cent go on to become bulimic. Incidentally we find that only 1 man for every 10 women suffer from eating disorders – they just help cause them by preferring slim, youthfully curvaceous women – or is it the women's magazines that do that?

It is a very sad thing that although we equate losing weight with ill health we are nonetheless drawn in by the contemporary myopia: the overvaluation of being slim. It is a sickness and preoccupation of our age and women in particular suffer from it.

Obviously the desire to be slender results in eating less, as well as eating foods especially designed to assuage hunger, which may be filled with all kinds of gut-adhering fillers, or even laxatives – so many diet foods contain these.

Inhibiting clothing, worn a size too small, also cramps intestinal activity and discourages its healthy muscular movements. With this obsession often comes an overwhelming desire to glut on all forbidden foods from time to time – what this does to the confused digestive system is anybody's guess but the results inevitably lead to digestive disorders of one kind or another.

This is bad enough if such problems coincide with the arrival of adulthood and the desire to be attractive in the contemporary way, but if they are also complexed with deep, psychological problems relating back to childhood, then the desire can become an obsession. Often colonic irrigationists see the results of all these categories, who come to them for the mistaken reason of using the treatment as a further means to help them lose weight.

EATING DISORDERS
AND COLONIC IRRIGATION

Anorexia nervosa and bulimia are eating disorders which often appear in adolescence or early adulthood and are very often complexed with a desire to rebel, common in all adolescents when establishing their own autonomy.

Unfortunately, in the case of these two eating disorders, the rebellion centres around food intake. It is a common parental pattern to try and get children to 'eat up' and very often rewards are given (of yet more food, usually the worst kind of treat food) if the regular meals are consumed. When the young person becomes aware of body shape and what they think of as desirable dimensions, they begin to slim, dieting not only for itself but also as a way of defying parents.

As body weight drops and brain chemistry begins to suffer from nutritional deficits so produced, a distorted view of themselves begins to take hold and anything more than bone-thin seems gross and overweight. At this stage, if not before, bowel problems start to emerge because of so little going through the system, and many of these by now severely affected young people (usually women) arrive at the door of the colonic irrigationist.

Not only has this given colonic irrigation a bad name as a treatment used by what is wrongly seen as self-indulgent young women who want to slim, but also the knowledge that they are not always turned away suggests collaboration by colonic therapists.

In talking to colonic therapists about this aspect of their work most find that gentle disuasion works much better than occasioning the sufferer another outright rejection. Also, there is some justification for doing a certain amount of cleansing work on a colon which is probably out of tone and may also be in need of clearing because of there being so little bulk in the diet.

Colonic irrigation can also be helpful in the case of eating and other psychological disorders because it is a very cathartic treatment, both physically and psychologically. The release of the bowel is often accompanied by a release of emotions and a recognition of what has been troubling the person undergoing the treatment.

Joan Osborne, a leading London colonic irrigationist of

many years' experience, both in America and England, expresses this aspect of her work thus: 'Psychologically today, some – most – people are burdened with deep seated problems. If they don't tell me I don't ask but often when the colonic begins to flow they begin to unburden themselves, and I say . . . was there ever a better time to throw all that away than down this tube?'

Osborne believes that people only lose what they need to lose in terms of weight.

> 'What we are ridding them of is excess poundage, poundage they don't need since it is accumulated waste. Slim people can have accumulated waste the same as fat people. I have one lady who is very thin and also very ill, and having a colonic helps her condition. She knows that but also worries about weight loss. I say, "who needs this kind of weight?" pointing to the sludge disappearing down the drain.'

Obviously Osborne recognizes there are limits in the case of psychologically-based eating disorders. No colonic irrigationist wishes to bestow on an already misunderstood profession an even worse reputation by treating those for whom treatment is inappropriate, if not debilitating.

In fact most colonic irrigationists come into this hands-on, no-holds-barred therapy because they have suffered themselves and their attitude is very much one of care and concern for their patients, over and above the call of professional duty. It has to be a very special person who can put clients at their ease under such circumstances.

Another top London therapist, Margie Finchell, humorously comments:

> 'people are not used to opening their bowels flat on a table with a

pipe up their bum and somebody watching to see what comes out. Once they overcome their reticence they realize that colonics are an exercise in letting go. It is the only therapy where you just have to let go and let somebody else take over. You can't be there all tight and wanting to be in charge. You have to relax and trust the other person. Just that exercise in letting go helps them to let go in other aspects of their life. That is why people change after a course of colonics.'

The treatment of people with weight and other problems is never simple and straightforward, but it may be that the fundamental approach of colonic hydrotherapy has a valuable role to play since it provides such extraordinarily apt facilities for unburdening, the physical paving the way for the psychological.

THE MULTIFACETED APPROACH TO STRESS

A mark of the new understanding of health is that no one treatment is expected to work out all a client's problems: human beings are complex creatures and their problems are correspondingly complex. Colonic therapists have recognized this and seldom use the therapy as an isolated treatment mode.

Jean Clark, President of the Colonic Irrigation Association says, 'Colonics are rarely used on their own. They are used in conjunction with other therapies and measures to create an environment for the body to balance itself.' Joan Osborne comments: 'I'm not saying colonics won't work on their own, but they'll be supported much better and you'll need a lot less of them if the combined approach is followed.' She adds: 'We teach clients to look after themselves.'

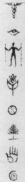

DE-STRESSING THE COLON: ADDITIONAL APPROACHES

Support therapies can include a wide range of alternative techniques, but the most effective would seem to be acupuncture (especially for bowel dysfunction), reflexology (which tones and balances all the internal muscular systems), aromatherapy (because of its powerfully relaxing effect on deep-seated body energy systems and its attendant lymph-drainage effect), hydrotherapy (for the same reasons), hypnotherapy (especially for eating disorders) and osteopathy and chiropractry (again because of their known ability to free up internal armoury). In fact in America, most colonic therapists practise in conjunction with chiropractry and usually advertize as chiropractors rather than as colonic irrigationists. Most people have a feeling for which therapy would suit them best; however, general advice would be to try several, and when in doubt, choose the therapist with whom greatest rapport has been felt.

EXERCISE FOR THE COLON

Exercise is vital if the colon is to be encouraged away from the sluggishness experienced in all muscles through leading a too-sedentary lifestyle. A half-an-hour's walk a day will 'get things going' and put the walker in a better frame of mind to deal with any stresses and problems. Learning a form of dancing is another tremendous releaser of stress as well as being excellent means of exercise. Keeping the stomach muscles taut but not tightened is all-important as otherwise abdominal contents tend to protrude and get out of place.

The new school of thought expressed by back experts contends that it is the stomach muscles that hold the mid-spine in place, not the other way round. The best and most obvious way of exercising stomach muscles is by

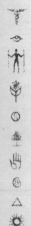

doing a type of sit up, but with certain constrictions.

HOW TO DO SAFER SIT-UPS

Begin slowly: do not attempt to actually sit up; just lie on your back with your knees bent and your hands on your thighs. Keeping your stomach pulled in, lift your head and shoulders off the ground no more than 45 degrees, sliding your hands up your thighs towards your knees as you do so. Then slowly slide them down as you lower your upper torso to the floor. Repeat up to eight times. Keep looking at the ceiling while doing this exercise.

DISEASE, THE ELDERLY, AND COLONICS

Since we tend to become more and more sedentary as life (or a disease state) progresses, there is a likelihood of developing atonic constipation, where the bowel has become so sluggish that it needs help to perform.

Provided there are no health reasons why colonics should not be performed, regular treatment can be of enormous help, removing wastes which might otherwise obstruct the healing processes. Obviously the use of colonic irrigation under such circumstances must be a matter between the person and their health advisor, their doctor.

SELF-HELP STRESS MEASURES[1]

(As published in the January 1994 issue of the *Colonic International Association Newsletter*.)

[1] Taken from an address given by Jim Robson, Primary Healthcare Coordinator, Newcastle & North Tyne Health Promotion. The text has also appeared in another newsletter published by the National Association for Colitis and Crohn's disease (NACC). See Useful Addresses

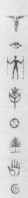

TALK IT OUT. Share it with someone else. Others will welcome your trust.

WRITE IT OUT. It is easier to see it in perspective when it is put on paper.

LAUGH IT OFF. Lighten it with humour. Be generous with smiles.

DISTANCE IT. Imagine a few years from now. How much will it matter then.

SHRUG IT OFF. Raise your shoulders, then drop them. Relax your body.

BALANCE IT. Consider the good consequences and feel glad about them.

BREATHE IT AWAY. Inhale deeply, exhale heavily a few times. Calm your thoughts.

CANCEL IT. Think positively, don't let the negative pull you down.

SORT IT OUT. List practical options, weigh, decide, then act.

EXAGGERATE IT. Picture the worst that could really happen. Is it really likely?

DELAY IT. Put aside 15 minutes for a worry session – leave it until then.

WIN THROUGH IT. Imagine yourself being successful and feel good about it.

WORK IT OUT. Do something physical. Clear your head, divert your energy.

HOLD IT. Say 'Stop', pause, think. Now take a fresh look.

REVERSE IT. Consider taking an opposite approach, explore alternatives.

ESCAPE IT. Notice something enjoyable around you. Get into the present.

Obviously, long-term deep complexes which reveal themselves in distortions in the unconscious nerve controls of the body are going to need more than prophylactics to sort them out, but body work, plus a willingness to apply the attention to resolving them, can begin the fascinating journey to recovery.

CASE HISTORIES
AND COMMENT

Does anyone want to talk about having colonic irrigation? Not so that you'd recognize them. But then a few years ago no one wanted to talk about orgasms and now that's almost commonplace. Times change. People adapt – then adopt the most unlikely new trends.

Until colonic irrigation loses its kinky image, everyone who has it will feel tainted with this stigma. In fact many more people would probably try the treatment, were it not for this. As it is, one has to be well along the rocky road of suffering from some bowel complaint or other before the pain actually overcomes the prejudice.

However, more and more articles are appearing about the therapy in the popular press and nearly everyone who writes about it tries it. Their experiences are remarkably similar. They emerge not only lighter in step but lighter in spirits too. Of course it's OK to try it if you are investigating something.

CRITICISMS

When criticisms do occur (apart from the physiological factors discussed in Chapter 3) they usually have a psychological angle, eg that such a treatment panders to neurotic (usually obsessive) tendencies. There is no doubt that psychological factors have been noted in patients attending gastro-enterological units by several researchers – so it would seem that the association is with certain kinds of bowel disorders rather than with colonic irrigation as such. In any case, one stigma which has thankfully been removed from the ill-health closet is that it is suspect if anything is psychological (mental) in origin. Now it is recognized that all diseases are psychological in origin: where the mind rules, the body follows. Or, as health expert and author Dr John Christopher said: 'There is really no incurable disease, only incurable people.'

Obviously a decision to try colonics must involve twin responsibilities: those of the therapist and those of the prospective patient. In the latter case, the obligation would seem to be that patients get to know as much about their bowel condition and the treatment they are envisaging as possible and that they choose their therapist carefully: in the former, there is a need to adhere rigorously to the code of ethics defined both by their own national association of colonic therapists, and in a broader sense, to those expressed in the code of conduct of organizations such as the British Complementary Medicine Association (or the American Complementary Association), which are clear about practitioners observing certain standards of care and skill and not treating people who will not benefit.

CASE HISTORY OVERVIEW

London-based Sister Allen, SRN, has been involved in colonic irrigation and other supportive therapies since the end of World War II, 1945.

At one time she had three treatment rooms and four changing cubicles on the go in her London consulting rooms. As is still the case in America, she used to practise under the umbrella of a well-known osteopathic practice.

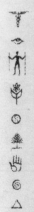

She later set up on her own (though still offering supportive therapies such as physiotherapy and steam cabinets – which she says were also very good for shifting and eliminating toxins) but the majority of her work was with colonics and 'encouraging the bowel to work on its own' through nutritional and other advice.

When she started she knew of one other woman who 'had an enormous practice in London', an ex-matron of a large London teaching hospital who had a discreet and 'celebrity-visited' practice in Marylebone High Street. (I actually lived in the adjacent apartment to this woman and often visited her socially, but never knew of her practice!)

According to Sister Allen, the few of her contemporaries who were interested in what today would be called holistic health concepts, all knew each other. Allen quotes Stanley Lief, founder of top health UK health hydro, Champneys, as saying, prophetically, 'in 100 years' time they'll all be thinking as we do.'

Allen had a lot of trouble with doctors who thought (and often openly expressed) the view that she was 'treading on their patch, taking bread from their mouths'. Nonetheless many sent their pre-op. patients to her to be washed out before bowel surgery or bowel X-rays – 'but never as a treatment mode: doctors don't reckon it helps the health at all'. She did attend one illustrious meeting of bowel surgeons and stood up and suggested that it might do some of their patients good to have their bowels cleansed of debris. She was met with stunned silence when she told them her patients got better and 'clearer-eyed'.

In fact Allen at 77 is an advertisement for her treatment, having as thick and healthy a head of hair as a young woman in her prime. Her clients, she said, 'were not run of mill, by no means a cross-section'. She classified them as being people who thought for themselves.

Did she get any kinky people? 'Remarkably few: but when I did they always came as a result of my advertisement in *The Times*. We could tell those immediately, because they appeared wearing the traditional bowler hat and furled umbrella. Of course not all those dressed like that were kinky, but one man did like being treated whilst wearing a lady's corset. Since he needed the treatment and gave no trouble whilst having it, we pandered to him.'

Sister Allen believes that the treatment proved itself over and over again in the many years of her practice – she retired 2–3 years ago which makes for nearly 50 years of giving colonics. She always used gravity machines but now she envies the capabilities of modern machines which are able to deliver oxygen or herbal additions.

She found that heavy meat eaters were the ones who needed her services the most – as for herself she keeps to a diet high in fresh fruit and 'plenty of roughage'. Because of her years of carefully watching her diet she needs very few colonics but has one if she needs it.

She used to be known (to her amusement) as 'the woman who does peculiar things to people'. One day she may be known as a health pioneer.

CASE HISTORY: COLITIS

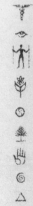

Doreen at 43 had despaired of overcoming her colitis as she had tried everything for the seven-year period of her illness, including steroid enemas, codeine phosphate and ingested steroids. At the time of her first colonic she had been off steroids for four weeks and had not only had continuous menstrual bleeding in that time but also had noted that her hair was falling out. She suffered regularly from thrush and had a travel phobia which meant she found it difficult to get into a car, so getting to her appointments was very difficult.

134

After her first colonic she was clear of her usual symptoms of passing blood and mucus for a week. During this period she agreed to change her diet dramatically, but noticed her symptoms returned one day when she ate a slice of wholemeal bread. It was discovered that she had a wheat intolerance which was not helped by the fact that her husband ran a café and so cakes and sandwiches were readily available for her.

By her third colonic, Doreen reported that she had got all her energy back and that her bowels had been fine for the two months between appointments. Doreen now says she has never felt so well and as long as she is fairly careful with her diet, her bowels now function normally.

COMMENT

It would be easy to attribute Doreen's improvement to diet only. Like so many of the complex illnesses around today, it is rare that one thing can be attributed to any improvement. What does seem likely is that clearing the colon enabled it to react more naturally to its allergen so that they could detect the wheat sensitivity which was behind her problem.

CASE HISTORY: VARICOSE VEINS

Glyn, 60, had suffered from varicose veins for most of his adult life, and when they were particularly bad eczema appeared around them as a complication as well.

Otherwise, he was in good health, except for the occasional migraine. After a course of colonics he began to notice an improvement in the eczema on the veins, also the veins themselves looked less angry. Now he uses the condition to let him know when he needs more treatment. Sometimes it clears up after two or three treatments, sometimes after only one. At the most he needs half a dozen treatments a year. Recently he has tried herbal colon cleanses which he feels are complementary to the colonics. He has passed old faecal material, sometimes black and with the consistency of hardened rubber. Now he feels more energetic than he felt in his fifties.

COMMENT

Glyn's improvement can be directly attributable to colonics as he was having no other treatment which could have been responsible for it. Like most people who feel better as a result of 'nature therapies', he now watches his diet more closely and has cut out meat and dairy products almost entirely. His need for colonics is decreasing.

CASE HISTORY: EMERGENCY BRAIN SURGERY

The husband of a colonic therapist had to have emergency brain surgery for an haemorrhage (aneurism). After the 5–6-hour surgery he recovered quickly and was out of intensive care in hours rather than days. There appeared to be no effects from the operation, no paralysis. Brian's health was good in any case, with a healthy diet and regular bowel movements, as many as 3–4 a day.

Suddenly, two months after surgery, he lost the use of his hand. The surgeon was mystified, arguing that if it had been a result of the operation he should have lost the use of his entire arm, not just the hand. He requested a number of tests but before agreeing to them, Brian was persuaded by his wife to have a seven-day cleanse (*see Chapter 4*). On the seventh day of the cleanse, black, rubbery, 'vulcanized' deposits started to come out of the colon, 'so black it was blue'. Brian decided to continue with the cleanse and this elimination went on until the tenth day. On the tenth day his hand started working perfectly.

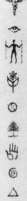

COMMENT

After encountering two case histories who described black, rubbery substances being eliminated from the bowel I telephoned a leading colon surgeon. He said he had never seen anything even remotely like it inside the bowel walls – 'it simply did not happen'. But I have no reason to doubt my case histories. There have also been photographs taken by colon therapists of hardened bowel contents, samples of which appear in Bernard Jensen's book, *Tissue Cleansing Through Bowel Management*. Who – or what – does one believe?

CASE HISTORY: CHRONIC CONSTIPATION

Jenny was 35 when she came to colonics having suffered from chronic constipation for ten years after experiencing an emotional breakdown. She moved her bowels perhaps once a week. It seemed that she had blanked out or 'forgotten' everything about her breakdown and felt she had internalized it. She was prompted to come to colonics because she had been reading that in Chinese medicine the colon is thought of as 'the second brain', also the place where we separate pure from impure thoughts. This bothered her.

Her stomach was very bloated and the therapist's perception of it was that it was 'very full'. During subsequent treatment she underwent a tremendous emotional, as well as physical release and started to recall details of her breakdown which she had entirely forgotten. Jenny has subsequently been able to deal with these issues in therapy. Her bowels are now moving regularly.

COMMENT

This case history is, so colonic therapists say, typical of the work they encounter. It is nothing for them to have patients (usually two weeks, even two months. The general consensus of any medical opinion such women are given is that the interval is all right so long as it is regular. But they rarely feel well.

After colonics and dietary advice most revert to once a day routines and say they feel considerably better.

CASE HISTORIES (2): RETAINED EXTRANEOUS MATERIAL

Vladek had had a barium meal in his twenties for a suspected gall bladder complaint. In his forties he decided to have a course of colonic therapy. During his third treatment he passed the white chalky substance which he had taken twenty years earlier.

Gordon has suffered from stomach and lymphatic cancer. After surgery the cancer returned so he decided not to follow traditional treatment any more but to follow the Gerson Therapy (*see Bibliography and Useful Addresses*). He also decided to have regular cleanses and it was during a treatment course (and whilst he was releasing copious amounts of black and hardened faeces) that he also passed a pull-ring from a can which he had swallowed as a child.

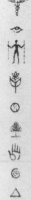

COMMENT

Therapists describe all sorts of effects coming from their clients. Some pass deposits of a certain colour which remind them, during the passing, of an illness they may have had, or a time when they were compelled to eat a diet which did not agree with them. The interesting aspect of this is that during the passing they often re-live and then are able to come to terms with the experience.

Some people are simply not helped by colonics. They do not pass anything of importance, some do not pass anything at all. Therapists have mixed opinions about this, but mainly they think such people are anal retentives, unable to 'let go'. Whatever the reason they are not ready for the treatment and may as well abandon it.

Others move on from colonics to self treatment with herbs and diet. Glyn has recently done this, preferring what he believes to be a more natural way of caring for the bowel. But he says that it was colonics that enabled him to understand the origin of his complaint, an unclean colon, and deal with it.

Possibly this is the sort of attitude that represents the consensus of opinion about the use of colon hydrotherapy – that it gets rid of past mistakes enabling a more natural healthcare to be embarked upon in the future.

PROTOCOL AND POLITICS

With a treatment such as colon hydrotherapy, which has struggled to survive since (1) the advent of freely-available laxatives and other drugs to prompt and control the colon, and (2) the abandoning of the procedure as a pre-operation measure in hospitals (where they now favour giving emetics through the nose) it is not surprising to find that what does remain of the profession is frequently under attack directly from orthodox medicine and indirectly from the drug companies which do their best to influence it. Drug companies are not interested in healthy colons, they are interested in selling laxatives for unhealthy colons.

In such a climate, a profession cannot be too careful about preserving the utmost integrity and quality within its ranks. Seven years ago, the Colonic International Association was formed in the UK for just that purpose – to establish firm standards of training and develop a protocol for invigilating and disciplining their members.

The President, Jean Clarke, says that this unfortunately sounds very bureaucratic, 'but as a practising therapist I have learnt how important it is to maintain and then improve standards in order to prevent the cowboys (and cowgirls) from getting a foothold in complementary medicine.'

She is aware that this is a critical time for alternative health. Admission to the EEC for its European members has meant that many therapies which may be traditionally understood in their own countries are having to meet general health requirements of the larger community. There is no room for error.

In America the same uneasy, changing picture exists. The CIA is now affiliated with their American counterpart, I-ACT, the USA-based International Association For Colon Therapy. This Association is five years old and has been formed at least in part to help combat moves to legislate against colonic therapists. (There is a move to do so in California which has been deferred for the time being.)

I-ACT is also anxious to establish standards and supervise anyone involved in Colonic Therapy (practitioners, manufacturers, distributors, other health care practitioners and even genuinely interested clients).

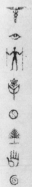

All this is very necessary if colonic irrigation is to effect a transition from being a little-known, often suspected, alternative treatment for improving bowel function to a well-known therapy such as acupuncture has become, or reflexology (also little known a decade or two ago). But an examination of the alternatives for this 'alternative treatment' surely justifies the efforts, they being laxatives and drugs to control but not cure, colon function, or the ultimate – bowel resection often necessitating colostomies.

The natural alternatives appear the more attractive proposition – diet, herbs, cleanses, therapeutic enemas. And of course a carefully-controlled amount of colonic irrigation.

REVIEW

A final review of the pros and cons of colonic irrigation might serve a useful purpose in this concluding chapter, leaving those who have read all or part of the text with a summary of salient points on both sides.

Here are the (said) benefits:

1   Makes the person more colon-aware and more willing to conserve and care for the colon. True.

2   Cleanses the colon of unwanted materials, some of them of long-standing, thus freeing up its musculature for more effective peristalsis and natural elimination. Confirmed by those who've had such problems, but whether this effect works for all is unproven.

3   Relaxes the musculature, may help to free adhesions, strictures and fibrotic attachments, thereby helping to unkink or untwist certain portions. Again, confirmation by both patients and therapists indicates the strong likelihood of this being so.

4   Relieves excess gas or bloating. Without question. I have had personal experience of this.

5   Is the ideal morning after the night before treatment – though hopefully it never should be overabused as such. I suspect Miss B's enormous practice in Marylebone was used by some for this 'porterhouse blue' purpose. NB: Porterhouse blue is an Oxford term used by dons, etc., to

describe those who love good cuts of meat and the good life in general, and pay for it with untimely strokes and heart attacks.

6   And finally one very underestimated benefit which I have personally experienced and observed: the treatment gets rid of silly hang-ups about the bowel and bowel function. It can't do otherwise – the evidence is before your very eyes!

Here are the main criticisms proferred (usually by the medical profession). And some comments about them.

1   The treatment may give pleasure (tch tch). NB: All the clients I have spoken to avow the only pleasure is relief of the burden which has been taken away.

2   Could cause intestinal perforation. Any internal invasion of the stomach area is in potential danger of doing this, as recent key-hole surgery misadventures have shown. The skill of the technician must be the key here. However, colonics experts assure me that this cannot happen – water is flowing in AND out at the same time, the patient is fully awake and (presumably) able to communicate and sense any real discomfort. Also pressure never goes beyond that exercised by 3 feet of gravity delivered through small tubes or 2 lbs of pressure per square inch (modern machines keep this down to less than 1 lb per square inch). US expert, Gary Lewkovitch, points out that a standard 2-qt enema can generate more pressure than this – as can stagnant intestinal gas. Certainly enemas produce more intestinal discomfort.

3   Delays vital treatment in some cases. This is exactly why

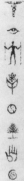

the better centres follow specific guidelines for screening patients. But it is worth commenting that painkillers could also delay vital treatment – and these can be purchased over the counter.

4   Colonics are habit-forming. Many people have found that just the opposite is true. Unlike enemas, laxatives, suppositories and similar, which undoubtedly are habit-forming, properly given colonic irrigation actually tones and conditions the bowel. But, like many other practices in life, colonics can be abused. Care is needed by therapist and potential patient. As with everything, moderation is the keynote.

5   Colonics irritate the intestinal lining. Not if given with properly treated water in which chlorine and other impurities have been screened out, and not when correct treatment modes are adhered to. Laxatives irritate far more. They even discolour the bowel lining.

6   Vital electrolytes and flora are washed out. This is a valid criticism but must be put into perspective. Firstly, there is the consideration that the cleansing will encourage the 'garden' to grow and support more successful crops of flora and generate better electrolyte activity in future. Secondly, implants and drinks given after treatment can counteract a large amount of this effect.

7   They don't work. How is it that this much-maligned, little-advertized treatment is therefore growing and growing? Over 90 per cent of all referrals come by word-of-mouth. What does limit the scope by which this treatment is used, regrettably, is its cost. So let's lobby that more natural, body-cleansing treatments like this one come back into the National Health, at least for a trial period. They might avoid

the cost of many expensive bowel operations – who knows until trials are done? Certainly they would encourage colon consciousness and complementary colon care.

NEW TRENDS IN COLON THERAPIES

A new understanding of the vital immune system of the body and the acknowledgement that 80 per cent of such activity may reside in the colon indicates that bowel therapies may become all-important in future in the control of infectious and degenerative diseases.

Research is already indicating such precepts. Pioneers such as Hans Peter Rusch, Arthur Becker, Hans Kolb and F.W. Hantel in Germany have been getting very positive results with rheumatic patients by repopulating the colon with advantageous flora, using at first highly diluted vaccines and finally live coli bacteria. These have seemed to establish more normal activity of the immune system and hence the rheumatic condition is controlled. F.W. Hantel has also successfully treated patients with colitis in this way. It is interesting to note that also mentioned as being instrumental in this new approach is enzyme therapy. There is a long way to go, but in the meantime an equivalent to the manufacturing industry's quality control seems necessary if colonic irrigation is to lose, once and for all, its many critics, some of them extremely well-respected.

Representative bodies of such therapists realize that trials must be done and research accomplished to test the claims of colonic irrigation. Meanwhile, a firm foot must be kept in the door of the alternative health scene in order to preserve a place for a treatment that may, in time and with care, be acknowledged as a useful adjunct in the prevention and improvement of all kinds of bowel conditions.

BIBLIOGRAPHY

* Denotes publication is a booklet.

Crook, William G. *The Yeast Connection* Biosocial Publications

Crook, William G. *The Yeast Connection Cookbook* Biosocial Publications

Cunnington, Ricky *Colonic Irrigation** Carnell Ltd, London, 1994

Durckheim, Karlfried Graf *Hara: The Vital Centre of Man* Mandala, Unwin, London 1988

Fasching, Rosina *The Tea Fungus Kombucha* Willhelm Elmsthaler Steyr, Weikang Ltd, Glasgow, 1987

Gerson, Dr Max *Cancer Therapy: Results of Fifty Cases* (Available in the UK from P.A. Faulkner, 57 Bridge Street, Pershore, Worcs. WR10 1AL and in the USA from PO Box 430, Bonita, Ca 02002.)

Grant, Doris & Joice Jean *Food Combining for Health* Thorsons, London, 1984

Gray, Robert *Colon Health Handbook* Emerald Publishing, Nevada, USA, 1990 (Also available from Robert Gray, see Useful Addresses.)

Janowitz, Henry D., MD *Your Gut Feelings: A Complete Guide to Living Better* OUP, Oxford, 1987

Jensen, Bernard *Tissue Cleansing Through Bowel Management* Bernard Jensen Enterprises, California, USA, 1981. (Also any other title by Jensen.)

Joice, Jean (see Grant, Doris)

Kettner, Joel (see Northover, John)

Leadbetter, C. W. *The Chakras* The Theosophical Publishing House, Illinois, USA, 1990

Lewkovich, Gary N., BC *Colonic Therapy** California, USA, 1986

Northover, John & Kettner, Joel *Bowel Cancer: The Facts* Oxford Paperbacks, Oxford, 1992

Painter, Neil S. *Diverticular Disease of the Colon* Keats Publishing, Connecticut, USA

Rauch, Erich, MD *Health Through Inner Body Cleansing* Haug Editions International, Brussels, 4th edition, 1993

Thomson, Leslie *The Healthy Human Gut: An Epitomised Version of James C. Thomson's Constipation and Our Civilisation,* Kingston Publications, Edinburgh, 1978

Trickett, Shirley *Irritable Bowel Syndrome and Diverticulosis* Thorsons, London, 1990

Truss, C. Orion, MD *The Missing Diagnosis*

de Vries, Jan *Stomach and Bowel Disorders* Mainstream Publishing, London, 1993

146   Walker, Norman *Colon Health: The Key to Vibrant Life* Norwalk Press, Arizona, USA, 1979. (And any other title by Norman Walker, eg *Become Younger* and *Fresh Vegetable and Fruit Juices*.)

Webster, David *Acidophilus and Colon Health* Nutri Books, Colorado, USA, 1991

Weinberger, Stanley *Healing Within* Weinberger Press California, USA, 1988

Winters, Jason *In Search of the Perfect Cleanse* Vinton Publishing Nevada, USA. (Also available from Revital – see Useful Addresses.)

Wright, Brian *Cleansing the Colon* Reasonhold Ltd, Green Library, Surrey, UK, 1985

Wunderlich, Ray C Jr, MD *The Friendly Bacteria* Keats Publishing, Connecticut, USA, 1988

USEFUL ADDRESSES

NUTRITIONAL AND HERBAL SUPPLIERS IN THE UK

Biocare, 54 Northfield Road, King's Norton, West Midlands
B30 1JH
Enzymes, sublingual vitamins, acidophilus and anti-candida
products.

Bioforce, Olympic Business Park, Dundonald, Strathclyde
KA2 9BE
Specialist herbs, eg for digestion.

C & G Food Supplies, 175 London Road, East Grinstead,
West Sussex RH19 1YY
Sublingual vitamins, skin brushes and anti-candida
products.

Larkhall Green Farm, 225 Putney Bridge Road, London
SW15 2PY
General and colon-cleansing supplies.

Natives Best, Freepost, PO Box 1, Tunbridge Wells,
Kent TN2 3EQ
Vitamins, amino acids and general supplies.

Revital, 35 High Road, Willesden, London NW10 2TE and
Victoria Arcade, London W1 (near Victoria Station)
Specialises in cleansing programmes, literature and
Eastern-based herbal preparations.

Rio Trading, 2 Eaton Place, Brighton, East Sussex BN2 1EH
Brazilian herbs including lapacho (pau d'arco).

Solgar, Solgar House, Chiltern Commerce Centre, Ashbridge
Road, Chesham, Buckinghamshire HP5 2PY
General vitamins and supplements. All products bottled in
glass.

Wholefood, 24 Paddington Street, London W1M 4DR
Organically grown produce, vitamins and herbal products,
including tea tree products.

NUTRITIONAL ADVISERS
AND SERVICES IN THE UK

Dunn Nutrition Centre, Downham's Lane, Milton Road,
Cambridge CB4 1JX
General

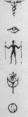

ION (Institute for Optimum Nutrition), Blades Court, Deodar
Road, London, SW15 2NU
Advice, general services, hair analysis.

Nutri Centre, The, (For address see The Hale Clinic under
Clinics and Health Centres in the UK below)
Tremendously wide variety of products, including rice
bran oil.

Nutrition Individual Diet Co., (To contact ring 01483 203555).

SPNT (Society for the Promotion of Nutritional Therapy), PO
Box 47, Heathfield, East Sussex TN21 8ZX

(For colonic therapists see separate list or contact the CIA –
Colonic International Association – address under Groups
and Organisations below)

Auchenkyle, Southwoods Road, Troon, Ayrshire KA19 7EL
General health (and bowel) problems.

Hale Clinic, The, 7 Park Crescent, London W1N 3HE
General alternative therapies, also colonics. Anti-candida
clinic.

ICHF (International Colon Hydrotherapy Foundation),
21 School Lane, Tolworth, Surrey.

ICHF Colon Hydrotherapy Clinic (Joan Osborne), 27 Warwick
Avenue, London W9 2PS

Richmond Clinic, The, 129 Sheen Road, Richmond, Surrey
TW9 1AY
General alternative therapies and nutritional screening/food
sensitivities, ozone therapy, candidiasis.

Wilson, Sally and Samantha, 56 Harley House, Marylebone
Road, London NW1 5HW
Alternative therapies, anti-candida, hypnotherapy for
anorexia and bulimia (Samantha).

USEFUL GROUPS
AND ORGANIZATIONS IN THE UK

Association of Reflexologists, 110 John Silkin Lane, London
SE8 5BE

Association of Systematic Kinesiology, 39 Browns Road,
Surbiton, Surrey KT5 8ST

BHMA (British Holistic Medical Association), 179 Gloucester Place, London NW1 3AP

British Society of Dowsers, Sycamore Barn, Tamley House, Hasingleigh, Ashford, Kent TN25 5HW

British Society of Nutritional Medicine, PO Box 3AP, London W1A 3AP

CIA (Colonic International Association), 16 England's Lane, London, NW3 4TG
Send SAE for list of therapists.

Council for Acupuncture, 179 Gloucester Place, London NW1 3AP

International Society of Professional Aromatherapists, The Annexe, Hinckley & District Hospital, Mount Road, Hinckley, Leicestershire LE10 1AG

National Institute of Medical Herbalists, Dept. H, 9 Palace Gate, Exeter, Devon EX1 1JA

National Register of Hypnotherapists and Psychotherapists, 12 Cross Street, Nelson, Lancashire BB9 7EN

ORGANIZATIONS AND PUBLICATIONS OFFERING ALTERNATIVE VIEWPOINTS IN THE UK

Dirty Medicine by Martin Walker, BM Box 8314, London WC1N 3XX

WDDTY (What Doctors Don't Tell You), 4 Wallace Road, London N1 2PG
Seasonal magazine. Contact at above address for subscriptions.

Chicago General Health Service, 1614 West Warren Boulevard, Chicago, Ill 60612

Colon Health Centre (Stanley Weinberger), PO Box 1013, Larkspur, Ca 94939
Supplier of DDS-1 acidophilus.

Forsyth, Dr Vanita, The Bowel Boutique, 1411 Fairground, Kingman, Az 86401

Gerson Natural Healing (Cancer) Clinic, PO Box 430, Bonita, Ca 02002

Healthexcel, Route 1, Box 495, Winthrop, Wa 98662
Anti-candida/parasite supplies and nutritional services

Holistic Horizons (Robert Gray), Box 2868, Oakland, Ca 94618–0068
Intestinal herbal formulas, books, etc.

I-ACT (Register of Colonic Hydrotherapists), 11739 Washington Boulevard, Los Angeles, Ca 90066

Jensen, Bernard, Route 1, Box 52, Escondido, Ca 92025
Intestinal/herbal treatments, books, etc.

Winters, Jason, 4055 S. Spencer Street, Suite 235, Las Vegas, Na 89109

Wood Institute, The, 2220 East Carlo, Bronson Memorial Highway, Suite 11, Kissemmee, Fl 34742

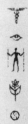

ORGANIZATIONS AND PUBLICATIONS
OFFERING ALTERNATIVE VIEWPOINTS
IN THE USA

Health & Healing edited by Dr Julian Whitaker, 7811 Montrose
Road, Potomac, Md 20854, USA
Seasonal magazine. Contact at above address for
subscriptions.

Racketeering in Medicine: The Suppression of Alternatives by
James P. Carter MD, Hampton Roads Publishing Co.,
891 Norfolk Square, Norfolk, Va 23502, USA

MAKERS OF COLON HYDROTHERAPY
EQUIPMENT IN THE UK AND THE USA

Aqua Hygiena & Aquazone Portable Machines, Jonathan
Bailey, 21 School Lane, Tolworth, Surbiton, Surrey
KT6 7Q8

Dotolo USA, 12555 Enterprise Boulevard, Largo, Fl 34643
(UK Distributors: Vindocto, 6–8 Market Place, Brigg, South
Humberside DN20 8HA)

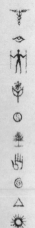

INDIVIDUAL COLONIC HYDROTHERAPISTS

This is by no means an exhaustive list of therapists to be found in this country. For a network of therapists in the UK contact either the Colonic International Association (For address see Useful Addresses, Useful Organizations and Groups in the UK) or the International Colonic Hydrotherapy Foundation (For address see Useful Addresses, Useful Organizations and Groups in the UK). For a list of therapists in the USA contact I-ACT (For address see Useful Addresses, Useful Organizations and Groups in the USA).

LONDON

Afra, Mrs C., 112b Northchurch Road, London N1. Tel: 0171 354 4136.

Chase-Hopkins, Mrs Mary, The Hale Clinic, 7 Park Crescent, London W1N 3HE. Tel: 0171 631 0156.

Clarke, Jean, 50A Morrish Road, Streatham, London SW2 4EG. Tel: 0181 671 7136.

Cohen, Mr Leor, Wellbeck Clinic, Flat B, 689 Finchley Road, Child's Hill, London NW2 2JN. Tel: 0171 435 0915.

Finchell, Mrs Margie, 5 Jacob's Well Mews, George Street, London W1H 5PD. Tel: 0171 935 5401 or 0171 624 5519.

Fitzgerald, Chryssey, The Fitzharding Clinic, 50 Beauchamp Place, Knightsbridge, London SW3. Apply in writing.

Gateley, Ursula, The Hale Clinic, 7 Park Crescent, London W1N 3HE. Tel: 0171 631 0156.

Grant, Mrs Anne-Lise, The Whole Health Clinic, 16 England's Lane, London NW3 4TG. Tel: 0171 722 9270.

Kahn, Mrs Adrienne, Violet Hill Studios, 6 Violet Hill, St John's Wood, London NW8 9EB or Neal's Yard Therapy Rooms, 2 Neal's Yard, Covent Garden, London WC2H 9DP. Tel: 0171 624 6101 or 0181 202 7151 (home).

Kirst, Ms Brigid, The South London Natural Health Centre, 7a Clapham Common South Side, London SW4 7AA or 5 Chipperfield Road, King's Langley, Hertfordshire WD4 9JB. Tel: 0171 720 8817, 01923 265151 or 0956 502342.

Lovrecic, Mr Borut, 26 Mulberry Way, South Woodford, London E18 1ED, or 140 Harley Street, London W1N 1 AH. Tel: 0181 530 8804 or 0171 486 4227.

Marshall, Sue, Wimbledon Clinic, 1 Evelyn Road, Wimbledon, London SW19. Tel: 0181 543 5477.

Monbiot, Katherine, The Hale Clinic, 7 Park Crescent, London W1N 3HE. Tel: 0171 631 0156.

Shaw, Ms Caroline, The Hale Clinic, 7 Park Crescent, London W1N 3HE. Tel: 0171 631 0156.

Stimson, Ms Roberta, The Naturopathic Practice, Dandelion Cottage, 14 Kendall Road, Isleworth, Middlesex TW7 6RA. Tel: 0181 568 9103.

Alder, Ms Maria, 82 Frances Road, Windsor, Berkshire SL4 3AJ. Tel: 01753 830470.

Batchelor, Mrs Elizabeth, High Spirit Lodge, 89 Edwin Road, Rainham, Kent ME8 0AE. Tel: 01634 233426.

Bailey, Mr Jonathan, 21 School Lane, Tolworth, Surrey KT6 7Q8. Tel: 0181 390 5402.

Blouet, Ms Anne, Harding House, 57 Upperton Gardens, Eastbourne, East Sussex BN21 2AF. Tel: 01323 412855.

Coburn, Ms D'Anne, 2 Bramley Nurseries, School Lane, Ashurstwood, West Sussex RH19 3QW. Tel: 01342 823650.

Eady, Ms Maria, 65 Buckingham Road, Brighton, East Sussex BN1 3RQ. Tel: 01273 323696.

Fairley, Ms Susan, 171 Sandown Road, Deal, Kent CT14 6NX. Tel: 01304 364879.

Neish, Ms Maureen, 21 Leafield Close, St John's, Woking, Surrey GU21 3HW. Tel: 01483 773958.

Warrington, Mr Michael, 6A Bedford Square, Brighton, East Sussex BN1 2PN. Tel: 01273 747132.

THE SOUTH

Piton, Ms Rachel, The Grove Natural Health Centre, 22 Grosvenor Road, Southampton S02 1RT. Tel: 01703 582245.

Siewert, Dr Milo, The Dorset Natural Health Clinic, 32A Wessex Road, Lower Parkstone, Poole, Dorset BH14 8BQ. Tel: 01202 717727.

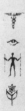

THE SOUTH WEST

Carter, Mrs J., Ringstead, Sutton Montis, Yeovil, Somerset
BA22 7AF. Tel: 01963 220449.

Groos, Mr Roger, Peggies, Beach Road, Woolacombe, Devon
EX34 7AE or First Floor, The Interior Shop, 6 Calenick Street,
Truro, Cornwall TR1 2EG. Tel: 01271 870436 or 01872 222265.

Noakes, Ms Pauline, 10 Eastfield Road, Westbury-on-Trym,
Bristol BS9 4AD. Tel: 01179 628302.

Wren, Ms Barbara, 5 Britton Close, Halburton, Nr Tiverton,
Devon EX16 7SH or Arcturus Centre, 47 Fore Street, Totnes,
Devon TQ9 5NJ. Tel: 01884 821761.

THE SOUTH MIDLANDS

Waterhouse, Ms Carole, 58 Knights Road, Blackbird Leys,
Oxford OX4 5DG. Tel: 01865 772384.

THE WEST MIDLANDS

McElroy, Mrs Helena, Clarendon College, 515 Hagley Road,
Birmingham B66 4AX. Tel: 0121 429 9191.

Pilling, Mr Daniel, 30 Lyndhurst Road, Rugby, Warwickshire
CV21 4HL. Tel: 01788 576366.

Trinder, Ms Jan E., The Creative Health Centre, 50A Warwick
Street, Leamington Spa, Warwickshire CV32 5JS.
Tel: 01926 316500. (See below also.)

Trinder, Ms Jan E., 19 West Road, Oakham, Leicestershire
LE15 6LT. Tel: 01572 724310.

THE NORTH EAST

Lambert, Ms Shirley Jay, The Caring Clinic, 35 Barkers Road,
Sheffield, Yorkshire S7 1SD. Tel: 01742 551345.

Lund, Mrs Margaret, Regal Chambers, 2nd Floor Suite,
22A Oxford Street, Harrogate, North Yorkshire HG1 1PU.
Tel: 01423 528533 or 01423 501927 (evenings).

Warwick, Ms Andrea, Hare & Hounds, 41 Teesway, Neasham,
Darlington DL21 1QT. Tel: 01325 721628.

THE NORTH WEST

Barbasch, Ms Audrey, 7 Rutland Road, Southport, Lancashire
PR8 6PB. Tel: 01704 530574.

Brown, Mr Richard, 70 The Avenue, Leigh, Lancashire
WN7 1ET. Tel: 01942 676617.

Neal, Mr Bill, 6 Bache Hill Estate, Upton, Cheshire CW2 1BR.
Tel: 01244 390953.

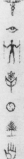

SCOTLAND

Bryce, Mr Eddie and Mrs Corinne, Fife Natural Therapies,
Albany Cottage Practice, Albany Street, Dunfermline, Fife
KY12 0Q7. Tel: 01383 732195.

PRINCIPLES OF
NUTRITIONAL THERAPY

LINDA LAZARIDES

Environmental pollutants and the use of antibiotics and other drugs cause changes in the body which can affect its ability to absorb and assimilate nutrients. Widespread nutritional deficiencies causing much chronic illness have resulted from this in our society. Nutritional therapists, complementary medicine practitioners working with special diets and vitamins, are often able to cure illnesses such as eczema, chronic fatigue, premenstrual syndrome, irritable bowel syndrome, hyperactivity and migraine.

This introductory guide explains:

- how deficiencies occur

- how nutritional therapy works

- which key illnesses the therapy can fight

Linda Lazarides is Director of the Society for the Promotion of Nutritional Therapy. She is a practising nutritional therapist with several years of working with a GP. She is an advisor to the Institute of Complementary Medicine and BACUP and is on the advisory panel of *Here's Health* magazine.

PRINCIPLES OF COLONIC IRRIGATION

PRINCIPLES OF AROMATHERAPY

CATHY HOPKINS

Interest in aromatherapy has grown massively over the last few years. Many people are realizing that the therapeutic properties of plants, contained in the oils extracted from them, can improve our health and well-being in many ways. This introductory guide explains:

This introductory guide explains:

- what aromatherapy is

- what its origins are

- what essential oils are

- how to use oils for health, beauty and relaxation

- how to find a practitioner

Cathy Hopkins is a long-time practitioner of aromatherapy and member of the International Federation of Aromatherapists. She is the author of the bestselling *The Joy of Aromatherapy*.

PRINCIPLES OF
NLP

JOSEPH O'CONNOR & IAN McDERMOTT

Neuro-Linguistic Programming (NLP) is the psychology of excellence. It is based on the practical skills that are used by all good communicators to obtain excellent results. These skills are invaluable for personal and professional development. This introductory guide explains:

- how to use it in your life personally, spiritually and professionally

- how to understand body language

- how to achieve excellence in everything that you do

Joseph O'Connor is a trainer, consultant and software designer. He is the author of the bestselling *Introducing NLP* and several other titles, including *Successful Selling with NLP* and *Training with NLP*.

Ian McDermott is a certified trainer with the Society of Neuro-Linguistic Programming. He is the Director of Training for International Teaching Seminars, the leading NLP training organization in the UK.